'Sally uses her humanity and her unique approach to life to enlighten people in how to approach and take charge of their cancer treatment choices. Lifting the lid on integrative medicine, Sally leads the way in utilising lifestyle and healing modalities to triumph over cancer.'

Patricia Peat, RGN, Dip Pall C Dip UTR, Founder of Cancer Options

'Sally bravely tells the story of her encounter with breast cancer – the physical and emotional difficulties, the psychological challenges and all the inherent risks to her public career. And we are all the richer for it.

This is Sally's journey through an inhospitable land tragically being visited by more and more of us every year. And, crucially, Sally is the one in the driving seat, the one deciding at each junction which is the right direction for her. Many of her decisions might not be right for you, but that is immaterial – they were the right ones for Sally, and she was at pains to gather the support and expertise she needed around her to empower her with sufficient choice and control to make them.

Supporting people with cancer in making their own choices is precisely the mission of Yes to Life, and so we are absolutely delighted that Sally has generously chosen to support the charity though sales of her book.'

Robin Daly, Chairman and Founder, Yes to Life

Actress, author and presenter Sally Farmiloe-Neville has worked in every field of the entertainment industry, and is currently senior presenter for B WELLTV and W6 STUDIOS and Editor in Chief of Hot Gossip magazine. She is also a member of MENSA. Sally lives in London with her husband and children, and is one of the city's top society hostesses and charity auctioneers. She is the British Chairman of Food Relief International and a Patron of Against Breast Cancer. Over the years she has raised hundreds of thousands of pounds for countless charities and worthwhile causes.

MY LEFT BOOB

A Cancer Diary

Sally Farmiloe-Neville

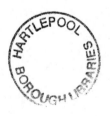

Book Guild Publishing
Sussex, England

First published in Great Britain in 2013 by
The Book Guild Ltd
The Werks
45 Church Road
Brighton, BN3 2BE

Typesetting in Fiesole by
YHT Ltd, London

Printed and bound in Great Britain by
4edge Limited, Hockey, Essex.

A catalogue record for this book is available from
The British Library.

ISBN 978 1 909716 03 2

To Adele Bloom, who suggested I write this book, to Dr Anna, Lady Brocklebank, for her kind advice at all hours, and to Jade, my reason for living.

Foreword by Professor Ian E. Smith, MD, FRCP, FRCPE

Consultant in Medical Oncology, Professor in Cancer Medicine, Head of the Breast Unit, Royal Marsden Hospital.

Treatment for breast cancer today is more effective than ever before, but it comes at a price. It can be long and difficult, and both physically and emotionally draining. This is the day-to-day story of how one remarkable woman coped, with cheerfulness, courage, good humour and great strength of spirit. It is packed with practical advice on all the many issues that inevitably arise during treatment, and her account of going through the rigours of chemotherapy will be of great interest not just to the public but to cancer doctors themselves. What comes through most strongly is the support of friends and family and of the dedicated nurses involved in her care. It is a story to warm the heart.

Medical Consultants

Professor Ian E Smith, MD, FRCP, FRCPE,
Consultant in Medical Oncology, Professor in Cancer
Medicine, Head of the Breast Unit, Royal Marsden Hospital.

Patricia Peat, RGN, Dip Pall C Dip UTR

Dr Miriam Dwek, BSc, PGDip (HE), PhD

Special Thanks and Acknowledgements

To all my loyal, supportive and patient family and friends
mentioned in this book and to everyone who kindly con-
tributed their personal stories.

To the following wonderful medics and staff at The Royal
Marsden, Chelsea:
Professor Ian Smith FRCP FRCPE, Dr N Turner PhD MRCP,
Dr M Parton MD MRCP (Consultant Medical Oncologists),
Geraldine and Andreas, Dr G Anandappa, Dr Tazia Irfan, Dr
Amna Sheri, Senior Outpatient Staff Nurses, Elena and Orla,
and all of Professor Smith's team.
Mr Gerald Gui MS MRCS FRCS, Miss A Agusti, Miss Toral
Gathani, Dr Matthew Yousif, Breast Care Nurses, Mel and
Vanda and all in the Breast Unit Surgical Team.
Clinical Research Nurse Yukie Kano.
Senior Nurses Sally and Sophie and Nurses Valerie, Beth,
Kathyrn, Mary and all in The Medical Day Unit.
Dr Fiona McManus (Anaesthetist) and Nurse Sandy and all
in Theatres.

Senior Staff Nurse Eleanor and Nurse Erika and all in the Day Surgery Unit.

Dr S Allen, Dr R Pope, Nancy, Lindsay and all in the Ultrasound Department.

Dr Gillian Ross, Dr Paolo De-Ieso, Linda, Mandy and Craig in Scanning, Jackie on Reception, Senior Staff Nurse Edith and Radiographers, Lucy, Di, Kay, Melissa, Punita, Rachel, Maxine, Faz, Kieran, Ben, Karen, Rosemarie and Lisa and all in the Radiotherapy Department.

Christina, Freddie and all in The Blood Room.

Catherine and all in Radiology.

Clinical Specialist Physiotherapy Kate Jones.

Paul and Gill in Hairdressing.

Rudi, Lisa and all in the Pharmacy.

Jackie and Biffa and all at The Friends of the Royal Marsden.

All of the staff on the Outpatients Reception, general Receptions and in the cafés.

Also to the following kind and helpful medics, health experts and advisors:

Dr Michael McKeown GP, Dr Jourdier GP, Dr Cole GP, Jodie, Crystal and Avery at Kynance Medical Centre.

Nurse Addie and the staff of Charing Cross Hospital.

The staff of Guy's Hospital.

The Harley Street Breast Clinic, Mr Michael Douek and Christina.

Mr Peter Cox and Peter Cox Nutrition.

Mr Robin Daly, Ms Sue De Cesare and all at Yes To Life.

Mrs Patricia Peat, RGN, Dip Pall C Dip UTR, Hayley and all at Cancer Options.

The Haven, Jill and all at Look Good... Feel Better.

Maggie's Cancer Caring Centre, London.
Emmanuel, Mary and all the District Nurses.
Dr Anna, Lady Brocklebank.
Dr Richard Hart.
Dr John Keet.
Mrs Pat Leathem, Dr Anthony Leathem, Mrs Wendy Taylor-Hill and all at Against Breast Cancer.
Dr Miriam Dwek and Dr Claire Robertson at Westminster University.
Mr David Goodman.
Mr Lucien Morgan and Miss Valerie Austin.
The Spiritual Healing Centre.
Lund Osler Dentistry
The Freiberger Dental Practice.
Mr Steven Smith.
The Spencer Clinic.

Publishing thanks:
To my wonderful team at Book Guild Publishing—
Carol, Joanna, Melanie and Louise.
Also to my own brilliant publicist and dear friend, Charlotte Ellis.

MONDAY 14TH MAY 2012:
'Off With Her Breast!'

'You have cancer in your left breast and we recommend a mastectomy.' Those were the words that turned my heart to stone that rainy May morning at London's Charing Cross Hospital. I was so shocked I burst into tears. Addie, the kindly blonde cancer nurse, rushed forward with a man-size box of Kleenex, and the doctor – who I later learned was a surgeon, so a 'Mrs' not a 'doctor' – said: 'Oh, was this not expected?'

Is it *ever* expected? No, I did not expect to get cancer. I was not that old, ate sensibly, didn't smoke, didn't drink too much and kept pretty fit with my tennis, cycling and workouts with weights. In fact I was a beauty, health and fitness writer and presenter, so I thought I knew a thing or two about it. However, my main income comes from playing glamorous acting roles and 'mature' modelling so I knew immediately that I would have to think about the aesthetic implications of losing a breast as well as the health side.

At the time, though, when I only had a ten-minute appointment, I was so numb that I couldn't think of anything to say. I just stared at the good-looking Asian lady doctor who was so calm about it all, and hoped I could bond with her. I can't remember what happened next. I was supposed to go to my tennis coaching but I couldn't face it so I stumbled home.

ADVICE: *If you can, always take a friend or family member with you to important consultations at hospitals. They can ask the sensible questions while you dissolve into hysterics!*

This all started in 2011. In 2004 I had had a letter from the NHS telling me that, now I was fifty (strange, I thought I was thirty nine!), I could have a free mammogram every three years. I knew these tests were a bit uncomfortable but I had had benign lumps in my breasts and under-arms before and decided to take advantage of the regular scans at my local Charing Cross Hospital. The first two had been fine but in 2011 they had spotted a little white speck on the left breast. I'd had a core biopsy, which wasn't painful, and then went in to see the consultant at Charing Cross to get the results. The radiologist hadn't turned up so the consultant, a Scottish gentleman, eventually saw me by myself, as with the other ladies that day. He told me the speck was a 'Level 3' risk and that I should come back for another test in one year's time. Level 3 sounded like intermediate to me and I thought maybe I should come back before that. I asked the doctor what the speck might be exactly – was it calcification maybe? But he didn't seem too sure and was in a bit of a hurry, so I just left.

A couple of weeks later I got a letter from Charing Cross Hospital stating that my 'speck' was 'Level 1'. That is the lowest risk category, so maybe an appointment in a year would be fine. But which was it? Level 3 as the doc had said at my results consultation, or Level 1 as they were now saying? I didn't get much joy ringing the hospital to find out, so my ever helpful and kind GP, Dr McKeown, wrote to them for me. I believe he had to send them a couple of letters but eventually they replied that it was only Level 1.

This sounded better – but why did the consultant tell me Level 3 before? Did he get it wrong because the radiologist was not there? I spoke to my dear friend, Dr Anna, Lady

Brocklebank, a specialist at St George's Hospital in south west London, and she said mistakes are often made and that I should go and get a second opinion privately at The Breast Clinic in Harley Street. I often think that I *was* Level 3 then and that if I *had* gone to the Breast Clinic at the time, I could have had further tests and might have averted disaster – 'spilled milk' and all that!

By this time, after all the fiddling about with the hospital letters, it was nearly summer 2011. The year before, I had returned to the stage, my first love, after my daughter Jade had left school. I had been rehearsing and playing in draughty theatres and travelling on the Underground, and I was constantly getting colds and coughs which would last for two weeks. Eventually, in July 2011, a cold developed into laryngitis and I had to cancel a performance for the first time in my acting career. This was a huge blow – I hated letting the theatrical company down, so I bit the bullet and went to a very expensive consultant in Harley Street. He sent me off to have several blood tests, again at vast expense, and then told me my immune system was low and put me on ten different supplements (fourteen pills) a day and a no wheat/no dairy diet. I immediately started this but got very irritable and weepy, shouting at taxi drivers and swearing at the other actors if they upstaged me – not good for my career or the general public. I rang the doctor and asked if I was getting withdrawal symptoms from my usual comfort foods. He said, 'Yes, of course – everyone gets that.' Well, he could have blooming well told me! I was more furious than ever but didn't want to take it out on him because he was a sweet old man. So I just did my own thing and *gradually* cut out wheat and dairy instead of doing it all at once.

3

I had lost confidence in that doctor but was lucky to re-meet nutritionist Peter Cox, who had been one of the contributors to my health and beauty book, *Sensual Pleasures And The Art Of Morphing Into A Health Goddess*, at a party given by my actress pal, *Ab Fab*'s Helen Lederer. He has kept me on the straight and narrow ever since through the immune system diet and now the Cancer Diet.

There are several books on the famous 'Cancer Diet' by various doctors and nutritionists and they do not all agree. I trusted the advice of my own experts and my special friend Adele, who firmly believes in optimum nutrition as the road to good health after a pre-cancerous scare when she was young. Adele kindly gave me all the various books on nutrition for cancer, got me off the dreaded microwave and stuck a list of 'good' and 'bad' foods on the fridge door where I could not miss it!

ADVICE: 'The Cancer Diet'. *The main points seem to be that too much sugar, fat and very processed foods are bad and fresh foods, especially fruit, vegetables and juiced 'smoothies' are good.*
This is what most experts seem to agree upon:
Brown rice is better than wheat as a 'staple'. Dairy is considered by some to be bad for breast cancer patients; soy and almond milk are better although there are some discrepancies about soy in general and the jury is out on this. Red wine is good, white bad. Dark chocolate is good and can be used as a 'treat' instead of milk chocolate. Manuka honey (and, I later discovered, agave syrup) can replace nasty white processed sugar. Dark vegetables are particularly good. Red meat should

be cut down – some experts say never eat it, some say only eat it once a week, some say twice a week is fine.

Green tea, wheat grass, walnuts, almonds, raw courgettes, turmeric, apricot kernels, broccoli, maitake mushrooms, Iscador (from mistletoe) and soursop (a South American fruit) are all supposed to be cancer fighters.

The general thinking is that alkaline foods are healthier and easier to digest than acid ones while a patient is on chemo and/or producing excess stomach acid due to the stress of the disease and treatments.

(Please refer to Patricia Peat's list of Acid and Alkaline Foods at the end of this book.)

The supplements and the diet worked and my colds would disappear after just a day or so. Because of all the blood tests and my new, healthy diet I presumed I was fit all over, breast and all. I hadn't requested any markers for cancer when I had my blood tests because the 'C' word had not been mentioned at that stage. That is why I didn't think I needed to get checked out at The Breast Clinic – and after my recent expensive visits to Harley Street (following previous family skirmishes with PPP and BUPA and having always been pretty healthy and careful about my lifestyle, I did not have any health insurance) I wasn't really in the mood for any more schlepping up there and wallet lightening!

ADVICE: Always ask about possible side-effects. Mistakes can be made privately as well as on the NHS and it's never good to go cold turkey on any new health regime as there may be unpleasant side-effects the doc hasn't warned you about. Don't be lazy and don't be cheap where your health is concerned. Your health is your most valuable commodity. Take out health insurance if you possibly can.

So that's why I hadn't had any more tests since the year before and why I was so shocked to find that I suddenly had a tumour big enough to warrant removing the whole breast. Granted my boob had been feeling a bit sore recently but I had put that down to the core biopsy, which had been very painful this time (should that have been a warning?). I had gone off to Palm Springs to visit my ex and best pal, Steve Rowland and his doggy, Mae Lynn, and had gone swimming every day in my padded, underwired pink bikini, boobies looking perky! I'd had occasional shooting pains but I'd had them in both breasts before and a doctor pal had said it could be just a touch of mastitis. (I later found out that women regularly get completely harmless pains in their breasts.) I did sometimes wonder what I would do if I had breast cancer but as I lounged in Stevie's pool under the brilliant California sun without a care in the world it just didn't seem possible.

I had gone out to visit Steve as soon as I had a break from the play I was doing at the time, *Carry On Brighton*, to cheer him up after his fiancée, Judy Lewis, had tragically died of a brain tumour. I had only met Judy on the phone but knew she was beautiful and famous, the 'love child' of Loretta Young and Clark Gable, and that her life had been snuffed out far too early. So I wasn't really thinking about my own small – or so I thought – problems.

Back to that unhappy day of my diagnosis... I had to tell my daughter Jade, who is the most precious person in my whole life. This was so hard. Poor Jade had lost her granny to cancer last year, her uncle to cancer four years before that, and her boyfriend had lost his mum to breast cancer two years earlier. So she equated cancer with death and instantly burst into tears when she heard her mumma had cancer. It is such a horrible word.

Those first few weeks after my first diagnosis were awful. Jade and I just lay on the sofa clinging to each other and mindlessly watching *The Kardashians* and *Two And A Half Men* (Charlie Sheen is my guilty pleasure but I doubt even the womanising Charlie would fancy a lady with only one bazooka!)

I never thought for a minute to doubt the diagnosis. I was to have a mastectomy with reconstruction at the same time: major surgery to remove the cancer followed by the reconstruction involving an implant, an expander in the bust which had to be pumped up regularly to stretch the skin slowly so it can accommodate the new, reconstructed breast, and muscle taken from my back to cover the implant, thus leaving another scar. All this because I am skinny and don't have enough flesh anywhere else on my body to make a new boob (although I believe a recon-struction with your own flesh is an even longer operation than the implant one). Then, inevitably, radiotherapy – and maybe the dreaded chemotherapy or pills. Those were dark days when I thought I might die because I didn't know if the cancer might have spread. I remembered the surgeon saying that they would do a sentinel lymph node biopsy at the time of surgery to see if it had spread to the lymph glands – the first place it spreads to from the breasts, apparently – but I wouldn't know until after they'd opened me up. However, my lack of knowledge was about to change...

Later that day I had rehearsals for the next run of *Carry on Brighton*. It was only a three-week run at my local theatre, therefore easy travelling, and I decided I should do it because the Charing Cross surgeon had said they wouldn't be able to operate for a few weeks. At rehearsals I took a big breath and told everybody my bad news and my decision. The writer/director Jackie Skarvellis and all the cast were wonderful and have been ever since.

The publicist suggested we go public with it immediately, before anybody else leaked it, which was bound to happen because I would have to tell so many people due to my work commitments. When something this dreadful happens you want to keep it to yourself and your family and close friends and when you work in the entertainment business you have the fear of never working again – especially if you are a middle-aged glamour girl about to take a lot of time off work and to lose an 'asset', as I was! So I said I would have to think about it very seriously. Ultimately they did give the story to the papers and that was the best thing that could have happened for me because so many people contacted me and gave me advice that would change everything.

That evening I was due to go to a film premiere and dinner with my friend Ruth Sherratt. I couldn't think of anything I wanted to do less but didn't want to let down Ruth, a lovely lady who was coming up from the country for the premiere. So I wriggled into an underwired bra and low-cut evening frock – how much longer would I be doing *that*? – and off I went with Robert Meah, my regular driver. In the event I had a lovely time. Ruth noticed I was very tense so I told her all and she was really sweet and insisted on treating me to a delicious dinner and a bottle of champagne at

Sheekey's seafood restaurant in Covent Garden, after which I felt much less pain.

And so to bed – on the worst day of my life – so far...

TUESDAY 15TH MAY:
A Test Appointment And Telling The Family

I made an appointment to have a smear test at my GP's tomorrow. When you're over 50 (which my mind often doesn't accept but my body obviously knows) you can get regular smear tests on the NHS as well as mammograms, plus tests for heart and strokes.

ADVICE: *Do all the tests – regularly – and have extra ones privately if any tests are inconclusive. Cancer can strike at any time. Look at me: I was quite fit and healthy and there is no history of breast cancer in my family.*

I rehearsed for the show, which took my mind off things. One of my fellow actors, Simon Brandon, was really worried about me so I was keeping it together for him and the whole company, to keep morale high.

I agreed to the 'going public' angle. After all, anything bad that's ever happened to me has always got into the papers, plus a few things that haven't actually happened to me too, so we might as well control it ourselves. Jackie decided to go with either the *Evening Standard* or the Richard Kay column in the *Mail* and we were all OK with that.

I then had a ring round to try to talk to someone who had actually had a mastectomy. I remembered Koo Stark had gone public when she had hers some years ago and thought she would be happy to talk about it but after many phone calls to mutual friends and stressing that it was something of an emergency, nobody could find her. I was a bit worried about her but happily someone later found her safe and sound.

Koo always said it was stress that had caused her cancer and I suddenly realised what a lot of stress I had had over the past year. Various people had owed me money, friends had let me down, the Inland Revenue were investigating me – vengefully, I thought – after I had refused to testify against my own accountant, and I had had to change my hairdresser after she failed to pay my charity for auction prizes that had been owing for months. (Other big-haired ladies, you will understand how traumatic it is to have to change your crimper! The good news is that that was how I found Steven Smith, a celebrity hairdresser who comes to your own home to weave his magic and now looks after Jade's gorgeous long blonde tresses and what's left of my hair after chemo.)

That evening we had a family dinner at a local gastro-pub restaurant, The Pear Tree, and I had to tell the rest of the family. My hubby, Jeremy, is pretty stoical and had been through all the cancer business – hospitals, doctors, treatments, diets, remedies – with his father when he was young and with his mother and brother-in-law in recent years, so he knew what to expect. Allie, my stepson, a budding chef, kindly promised to make me some lovely meals while I recuperated after my op. I told my brother, Crock, who was shocked because I had always been so healthy, and I am afraid I left him to tell my sister-in-law. The second hardest person to tell, after Jade, was my 'step-in' daughter Kat (she calls me her 'step-in' mum, because I stepped in and she came to live with us when her mother Marilyn, a close friend, died and her father remarried.) Marilyn had survived breast cancer, a lumpectomy, but sadly went on to die of something else and I knew Kat must be reminded of what had happened to her dear mum.

The Pear Tree restaurant is next door to the Charing Cross Hospital and I stared at that big building looming over us and pondered my fate. Both Jade and I had been treated well and kindly in their A&E department and my brother had spent several months there after an accident. I had dark thoughts, guzzled more Prosecco than usual and wondered if this trauma would turn me into an alcoholic!

WEDNESDAY 16TH MAY:
'Coming Out' About Cancer

I had my smear test with the lady doc at my GP's, at the same time discussing my breast cancer briefly and being assured that in a couple of years' time I would be old enough to have free colon and bowel tests as well. I feel that, now I am a cancer sufferer, I must really look after myself for the rest of my life and might as well have all the tests as long as they are not dangerous in any way (I think the jury's still out about radiation from mammograms but mams are clearly a necessary evil – if indeed they are at all evil.)

I remembered that my dear friend Georgina Bruni, who had survived breast cancer, had later tragically died of ovarian cancer and so I was very fearful. Georgina had been like a big sister to me, founded Hot Gossip, the online magazine which I've kept going in her memory, and always let me benefit my various charities at the networking club nights she ran. I knew how much poor Georgina had suffered at the end, God rest her soul.

In fact I had various friends who had had cancer but many did not want to discuss it and I had to respect that and not ask them for advice. I remember one special friend who had been so afraid of being seen at The Marsden in a wheelchair, the poor girl.

I totally understand why some people don't want people to know they have cancer because they feel it will affect their work adversely and they will lose bookings. One friend of mine who had breast cancer drove herself out to the Sutton branch of the Marsden every day to have radiotherapy after her lumpectomy so that nobody would spot her at the Chelsea Marsden. I felt so sad for her when she told me. It is not right that people should judge you badly because you have cancer – it's not shameful, just the ailment of our modern age. But despite my misgivings, I was about to find out just how much wonderful support I would get as a cancer sufferer...

In the event, Jackie and co. had given the story about my cancer to the Richard Kay column at the *Daily Mail*, which was fine because it's a classy column and Richard and his cohorts, Helen Minsky and John McEntee, have always been decent to me (unlike in the old days of Richard's predecessor, Nigel Dempster, who definitely lost me a boyfriend or two with his dreaded revelations – we all trembled in our boots when we knew he'd got something on us!). The story came out today and Richard had treated it in a very positive way, mentioning how we were all 'carrying on' with entertaining the troops in spite of all the disasters that had befallen the production, what with Jackie losing her surrogate mum and our leading man's mum having a stroke as well as my cancer. A dreadful time for them as well as me.

A lot of people contacted me immediately and asked me all about it. When I revealed that I had a cancerous lump and had to have a mastectomy but that there had been a bit of a mess-up in the diagnosis last year, they all said the same thing: get a second opinion! I had already discussed it with my publicist and close friend Charlotte Ellis and she had wondered why I couldn't just have a lumpectomy, which is a minor operation. Then Tatiana von Saxe Wilson, another close friend, rang me. 'You must go to the Royal Marsden immediately and see the wonderful Professor Ian Smith,' she said, and kindly got the ball rolling.

I attended rehearsals for the show then raced off to get 'Jinny lashed' in the West End. 'Jinny lashing' is not some weird *Fifty Shades of Grey* type of erotic thrashing but a lash extension treatment where a beautician sticks gorgeous, sweeping, feathery, semi-permanent eyelashes onto your natural ones à la Katie Price and Cheryl Cole. I had been wearing fake lashes for my part of 'Fenella', a glam cabaret singer who was definitely a huge eyelash gal, but I was crying so much at the moment (from fear and self pity, because I wasn't really in pain, just a bit of discomfort from the core biopsy – in fact they say that cancer doesn't hurt and that's why you need tests to find it) that I thought I'd never keep the lashes on! So Mr Cho, the technician at Jinny, applied some extra long, curly permanent lashes, which made me feel very Fenella!

I told Sarah, the manageress, about my diagnosis and that I was worried I might have to have chemo at some stage. She said not to worry, they can stick lashes onto your skin, top and bottom, if all your own lashes fall out. Oh my God! I hadn't thought of that – you lose your lashes and your brows as well as your hair with chemo – cue for fresh tears!

That evening I went to my pal Lalla's party at the Millennium Hotel with my bro and my close friend, Adele, who has a jewellery business and lives with us part time when she is working 'down South'. All my friends were full of advice and kind words for me. Annie, the Millennium PR lady, reminded me that one of our mutual friends had had a completely successful double mastectomy with top surgeon Mr Gui at the Marsden, and that's where I should go. I later spoke to our friend at length and she told me she had had to have mastectomies on both sides at different times, the poor thing, but that she was delighted with the eventual result. She hadn't had to have any chemo or radiotherapy, thank goodness, and said she was now completely clear and that her new boobs looked much better than her old ones! I started to feel a bit more cheerful. If I can just get what seems to be the Marsden 'dream team' of Professor Smith (oncologist) and Mr Gui (surgeon) I will be in the best hands.

THURSDAY 17TH MAY:
Frox And An Ex

I collected my girlfriend Rose-Marie, 'the Oirish singer who dossn't need a microphorn', as I always call her in my cod Irish, and we drove out to Borehamwood to Dynasty, a glitzy, evening dress label where Rose-Marie's friend Vivien King-Lawless was in charge of loaning out frocks to celebs for red carpet events. R-M is a platinum-selling singer and a big celebrity, and I am of course a very important, Z-list cel-ebutt! We left with armfuls of gorgeous, colourful frock-ettes for our next few parties. I was careful to clock the kaftans while there as I felt I would shortly be needing one to cover my left boob rather than show it off!

I put on one of the dresses – a bright red one – which instantly cheered me up, and R-M, Viv and I sped off to a fashion show by Colcci, the label which is co-endorsed by naughty Ashton Kutcher. Sadly he wasn't in evidence although Sophie Anderton was, and I couldn't help noticing how stunning her boobs looked, though not that big. After my chats yesterday I know that many ladies have their other boob cut down to the same size as the mastectomied one so that they still look symmetrical, and I was prepared for that if necessary.

There was a photographer there that I've always found extremely irritating and he didn't fail me tonight, wandering over and talking about some poor celeb who had just died of cancer and saying brightly, 'Lots of people are dying of cancer these days, aren't they?' R-M, Viv and I all glared at him but he just smiled back benignly. I am sure he hadn't seen my mention in the paper, it was just unfortunate. The girls reminded me that I needed to keep away from stressful and negative people and situations now that I have cancer. OK, cool; 'Smile and wave, smile and wave'!

But I was really rattled by this incident and, as we drove off to Motcombs, a Belgravia bar, for a nightcap, I rang Enzo, my ex toyboy from my unmarried days, and asked him to meet us there, where I proceeded to tell him all as I got royally smashed. Although twelve years younger than me, he is much wiser and more practical than *moi* and I have often turned to him for advice over the years. Enzo being Enzo swore that he would always worship my body even after the mastectomy, then never phoned me for three months (I remember why I didn't marry him now!) But the flattery was helpful, God bless him.

FRIDAY 18th MAY:
Referral To The Marsden And A Happy Ending For A Charing Cross Patient

I had another appointment with the lady surgeon and the nice nurse at the Charing Cross Hospital. In the meantime I had been copied in on a letter she had sent to my GP. It said:

'Histology showed a Grade 2 invasive ductal carcinoma with intermediate grade DCIS. The tumour was oestrogen, progesterone and HER2 negative. Her case was discussed in our Multidisciplinary Team Meeting, and the recommendation was for a mastectomy and sentinel node biopsy.'

It was all gibberish to my unmedical mind but I cut it out and stuck it in my diary so that I could discuss it with doctors, experts and, importantly, other breast cancer patients, in the future.

When they had shown me the core biopsy X-ray, the tumour had looked quite small and I knew that I must pluck up the courage to ask for a second opinion about having a mastectomy. I felt dreadful because I didn't like to question medical knowledge and upset the Charing Cross ladies, but after the mix-up with the tests the previous year and everything my friends had been telling me, I had to. Tatiana had told me I would need a referral to see Professor Smith, so I asked if I could please be referred to him and Mr Gui at the Royal Marsden. It was much easier than I expected; the surgeon immediately agreed and I was on my way to a brighter future.

In the meantime the Evening Standard had published a news item on my unhappy state (written kindly) and lots of my friends had been getting in touch to cheer me up and tell me their stories. One chap, whom I knew from volunteer fundraising for The Bob Champion Cancer Trust, said he had had a successful prostate cancer operation and had stuck a 'post it' note on his wotsit for his surgeon! Great – maybe I will leave one on my boob when the time comes.

My good friend, the actress Debbie Arnold, had put me in touch with another nice actress pal of hers who had had a successful mastectomy at the Charing Cross. Although this lady had had a similar problem to me with the same male consultant who had been rather unhelpful, she had been very pleased with her eventual operation. She said they had taken flesh from her tummy to reconstruct, then taken the other breast down to the same size to make her bust line symmetrical. So she had had a free tummy tuck, reconstruction and breast reduction all on the NHS! Her career had not suffered and she was now in a hit TV show. I so admired her, as I do all mastectomy patients, for what she had gone through and she admitted that she had had some very dark days. Hers was an inspiring story and I was so glad to hear she was working more than ever with her gorgeous new figure.

I had explained to the Charing Cross surgeon that I too really *needed* to work and earn plenty of money so that I could look after my family and myself in the manner to which we wanted to be accustomed! And I had also explained that I only needed my cleavage for my work as a so-called glam actress and mature model, not the left out-side bit of my breast where the tumour was. I didn't really mind having a little dent in there as no one really sees that bit in clothes. The only people who might see me undressed are my family and I hope they love me with all my imperfections.

However the Charing Cross lady didn't really 'get' that and the fact that I didn't want to be off work for too long, if humanly possible. I was a middle-aged housewife and mother in a highly competitive freelance business and didn't want to be forgotten... the old thing about losing work. I wondered if the docs at the Marsden would get it.

WEDNESDAY 30TH MAY:
The Royal Marsden

Yes, they do seem to get it at the Marsden. The hospital is wonderful, so calm and peaceful and well-furbished, like a private hospital, and they seem to have plenty of staff. I would never knock my local, Charing Cross Hospital, and have since campaigned against closing its A&E, but all the big hospitals are so huge, rabbit-warrenny and scary, especially with all those poor people in A&E. The Marsden is quite different. I went to the Rapid Diagnostic and Assessment Centre (RDAC) next to the modern looking

Wallace Wing of the hospital on Dovehouse Street, a side street away from the imposing, orange-brick Fulham Road front entrance of the grand old hospital, which I later learned was founded in 1851. I presume the RDAC centre is called 'rapid' because it deals with more urgent cases – but then I guess all cancer is urgent.

Professor Smith and Mr Gui were away but I saw a very nice breast consultant from Mr Gui's team who told me I should be able to have a 'wide local excision' instead of a mastectomy. This meant that they would remove the tumour, plus a margin round it to mop up any floating bad cells.

The bad news was that as my oestrogen, progesterone and HER2 were all more or less negative – making me 'triple negative' (as apparently 20% of breast cancer cases are) – I wouldn't respond to the usual pills, Tamoxifen and Herceptin, and would probably have to have chemo as well as radiotherapy afterwards. My blood ran cold. I have always been full of admiration for my friends and relations who had been through chemotherapy, that frightening, debilitating, treatment with dreadful side-effects, but I simply didn't know how I could be brave enough to face it myself.

The doc also said I should come off my HRT at this stage and that I might get my hormonal symptoms back. 'Oh no!' I thought. I was so irritable and weepy before going on HRT. Now I have something rather more important to worry about and am weeping every day anyway! But this doctor said that I would have an ultrasound test to see if the cancer had reached my lymph nodes, so at last I would know if it had spread – my big fear. I hadn't been offered this before surgery at the other hospital and was positively joyous.

I spent thirty minutes with the doctor then another thirty minutes with kind breast nurse Melanie, who explained many things to me about my possible surgery and treatment. It was so nice not to have time restraints – I just never had time to ask anything at the other hospital where each patient is allotted ten minutes. Thank goodness the Marsden had been founded for cancer patients and given a Royal Warrant.

Nurse Mel explained that a 'wide local excision' was a lumpectomy – also called 'breast conserving surgery' – and that it was minor surgery instead of major, like a mastectomy. She also said that I could transfer my care to the Marsden. It was slightly further away for me but I know that patients came from all over the country to this special centre of excellence.

In the last few days we had opened successfully in *Carry On Brighton* at our latest venue, The Draycott Theatre, and a lady called Patience (whom I was sadly never able to track down) left a package for me at the theatre. It contained a cancer book she had written and a letter explaining that 'You are *not* stuffed if you have more than one cancer' (which I had presumed and mentioned in my *Evening Standard* interview) and that she was happily bashing on, living with five cancers. What an amazing lady – I hope she will contact me again one day. So in general I am feeling much more positive. I still have discomfort in my left breast after the core biopsy, especially when wearing the triple-padded, underwired bra which was part of my onstage 'Fenella' cozzi, and I know I need surgery as soon as possible after the play finishes – but it will be so much better to have minor rather than major surgery if I can.

SATURDAY 2ND JUNE:
The Hurlingham And Madame Claude's

My close friend Adele Bloom was staying again and we got spruced up and trotted off to a glam car event at my club, The Hurlingham. We had a nice lunch and admired the Ferraris and Maseratis on the club's beautifully manicured green lawns. All seemed well with the world. Then my friends Arthur and James introduced us to a feisty lady magazine editor and we had an interesting chat. She knew about my problem and said, 'Oh well, if you do have to have a mastectomy, why bother with reconstruction?' A valid point if I didn't make my money from being glamorous as I don't think for one moment I get booked for my IQ!

If I had a double mastectomy that would be one thing, I would just be a flat-chested female. But to have one big one and one flat one? I can't see it being a popular look for my sort of work! I suddenly had a very non-PC flashback to the seventies when I had worked with a beautiful, one-armed model called Rosemary. She had not got a lot of modelling work with her disability, the poor girl, but had later become a big hit at the salon of Madame Claude, the famous Paris madame! God bless her wherever she is now. It's funny the things you remember when your life gets turned upside down.

WEDNESDAY 6TH JUNE:
Chemo Before Surgery

Breast nurse Mel from the Marsden rang to say that in the last meeting the docs had discussed giving me chemo *before* surgery to try to reduce the tumour and thus make the lumpectomy easier and give a more aesthetic result, i.e. a smaller dent in my boob. She said I would not need another core biopsy, which was good news as I was still sore from the original one in April.

ADVICE: Mel said: 'Do not touch your lump!' It's very tempting to keep feeling it now I know where it is but I know this will aggravate the tumour and make it sore. Obviously the reason it's still hurting me at the moment is because of the tests and examinations. I had now finished the final run of Carry On Brighton so did not have to wear a constricting bra and cozzi any longer and found that a soft sports bra was the most comfortable.

THURSDAY 7TH JUNE:
'Not Dead Yet' – And Nor Am I!

I had been carrying on my social life as normal, cheering myself up and looking and feeling quite well although a bit tired, which was probably from stress. Today I went down to the Grand Hotel in Brighton with my promo film-making partner Kazzy, to interview the famous thriller writer Peter James at the launch of his latest crime novel, *Not Dead Yet*. Peter is a long-time friend and a film producer, as well as a bestselling author. I modelled for his mother Cornelia James, glovemaker to The Queen, (although I tended to model dresses for her rather than Her Maj's gloves!) and had appeared as Francesca, a lingerie model, in one of his films, the iconic *Spanish Fly*. I was proud to be the friend of such a superstar (Jade calls Peter a 'legend') and was happy to be interviewing him for a promo film, as I had done before. My Brighton friend Mike Williams, with whom I'd stayed when appearing in *Carry On Brighton* in Brighton, came along as well and we had a jolly time as well as working.

The extraordinary thing was that Peter's PR guru, Tony, told me how 'absolutely radiant' I was looking. Obviously he didn't know and was just being nice. I guess one probably looks quite normal until actually starting the cancer treatment; I think in the old days before early detection we all probably carried on with cancer inside us for ages and then one day died. Well, that is not going to happen to me.

I later met a man who didn't know me and my situation, and he told me all about his wife's ovarian cancer; it was actually uplifting because she was doing well and I know that ovarian is a nasty one.

FRIDAY 8TH JUNE:
Missed My Surgery Date

My doctor friend Anna Brocklebank rang to kindly reiterate that her hubby John and she would be delighted to have me to stay at their beautiful house in the country, complete with *tous conforts* and a swimming pool, after my op. I love Anna's vibrant company, so that will be great.

She also reminded me that I had promised her I would make an appointment with the Harley Street Breast Clinic, which she had originally recommended to me the previous year, so I got on the phone and did so.

Then Addie, the breast nurse from the Charing Cross, rang me to say that they had a date for my surgery the following week but hadn't been able to get me on the phone. I burst into tears when I heard this. I don't know why, because I am pretty sure now that I don't need a mastectomy and therefore won't be operated on at the Charing Cross. I guess it was just the strain of everything. Addie was very sweet and told me that the surgeon was very experienced and had done loads of these mastectomies with reconstructions but more and more now I was hoping to avoid that huge operation.

Later that night I lay on my stomach and thought how soft my dear little left boob felt and how it would probably feel rock solid after the reconstructive mastectomy. I've never really rated my boobs and always thought my legs and bum were my better features. My bust is very asymmetrical, with my poor, diseased left one being half a size smaller than my right one (now if my *right* one had been the diseased one, they might have looked more even after surgery!). But it's a sad fact of life that you don't really miss things till they're gone and I just knew I would miss my old friend on the left if I let them lop it off. My boobs and I have been through a lot together – not just pregnancy and breastfeeding but being squeezed and hoisted up into so many costumes and frocks for work. Not to mention, of course, all of their good work on the red carpet at social events. One of my most fun and longest-running endorsements had been for an evening dress company, FanniAnn, who liked me to be snapped in their gorgeous gowns at the BAFTAS and so on. Plus I had endorsed a health food supplement that made your breasts bloom (it really worked well but sadly made one's body bloom everywhere else as well!) Happy days.

SUNDAY 10TH JUNE:
Last Hurrah For My Left Boob?

I compered a charity event in aid of Moorfields Eye Hospital for music impresario Henry Hadaway's 70th birthday and had a hoot trying to conduct an auction with Bobby Davro and Kenny Lynch. Frock-wise I was wearing a very low-cut, sparkly number from Dynasty and debated with my pals Adele, Rose-Marie and Vivien if this would be the last time my boobs would be out for *OK! Magazine!*

TUESDAY 12TH JUNE:
Another 'Second Opinion'

I finally went to The Harley Street Breast Clinic, as I should have done last year, for my private second opinion. I really wanted to be treated at the Marsden if possible but thought that I might as well follow Anna's advice and see what the private clinic advised while I waited for my Marsden surgeon of choice, Mr Gui, to return from abroad. There is no shame in being a bit of a 'health tourist' and shopping around for your medical treatment when it is something so important and especially if, like me, you do not entirely trust your first opinion.

After giving me an examination, and looking at the histology, the Breast Clinic surgeon also told me that I could probably get away with the smaller operation, the lumpectomy. I asked him how soon I needed to get it done – was it true that cancer spread every six weeks? No, he said, cancer doesn't necessarily grow every six weeks, but one shouldn't leave surgery or treatment a moment longer than necessary after diagnosis. Although I had actually been given my diagnosis on May 14th, I had been diagnosed a month earlier, but I had been away on hols at Steve's, and the Charing Cross Breast Care unit hadn't been able to fit me in to give me the news until two weeks after my return.

ADVICE: *Private health care is different – you do seem to get results more quickly. Our British NHS is wonderful in many ways but it might be good to keep up your health insurance if you can afford it.*

The Breast Clinic surgeon told me that at 57, I was 'young' (what?!) to go through cancer and I should get a good result. The bad news was that because of being 'triple negative (a fact that would return to haunt me), I would probably have to have both chemo and radiotherapy whether I had a mastectomy or a lumpectomy. It really was a no-brainer. Why on earth should I have that great big major surgery if the minor operation would be just as successful and I would have to have chemo and radio therapy with either operation? The surgeon also said I should probably have chemo *before* surgery to shrink the tumour and make it more easily operable. I was pleased that a second surgeon thought I didn't necessarily need a mastectomy.

WEDNESDAY 13TH JUNE:
Second Visit To The Marsden

I had my second visit to Mr Gui's clinic in the RDAC (Rapid Diagnostic & Assessment Centre) building at the Marsden. I'd promised Jade she could come with me this time but I chickened out and tried to sneak out without her! However she came running after me and was so upset I had to take her. When we arrived, I discovered there are seven special Marsden-only parking bays outside the hospital and I was able to get one for Violet, my beloved violet-coloured convertible. This was great news as parking in London can be an extremely stressful business. However, I realise that some people come from miles around to be treated at the Marsden and some patients are there all day so I had better be decent and get back 'on me bike' when I can!

This time I was measured and weighed and, although my height was still 5ft 7ins, my weight was over eight-and-a-half stone on the hospital scales, as opposed to under eight on the home ones. Even taking clothes and shoes into account I realised the scales at home were obviously wrong – no problem for Jade and me who are both very light but Jeremy was most annoyed when I informed him later!

I finally met the legendary Mr Gerald Gui, whom so many former patients had recommended to me. He is super efficient and immaculate but both Jade and I detected great compassion behind his business-like exterior. Mr Gui said I would have an ultrasound next to get a closer look at my tumour and check the lymph glands. This was music to my ears, as I had never been offered this test at the other hospital. Things were moving at this one. We discussed the possibility of chemotherapy before surgery to shrink the tumour, and radiotherapy afterwards. Mr Gui said that people respond differently to chemo, so he couldn't be sure exactly how much and when I would feel the nasty side-effects of this dreaded treatment but that I would have three weeks between each chemo treatment to recover. He said luckily my tumour had been picked up early so was still isolated, which was also good news.

Discussing my tumour with the surgeon who would operate on me, and the breast care nurse, Orla, seemed to bring it home to poor Jade, who was visibly upset – which of course upset me. Mr Gui and nurse Orla were very kind but we ended up snivelling away. However, Jade wants to be involved in all my important decisions and I must respect that.

My doctor friend Anna had suggested I asked for a CT scan of my whole body just in case there were any other nasties, especially in my bones. I asked nurse Orla about this but she explained that they did not usually do this any more as, if breast cancer had spread it would always travel to the lymph nodes first, and the ultrasound would detect anything there.

Mr Gui said that if I wanted to be transferred officially to the Marsden for my care, I would need to get my GP to refer me. I really, really wanted to be treated there where they were so efficient and kind, but I knew I would feel guilty about leaving the Charing Cross where nurse Addie had also been so sweet.

Later that day I spoke to my long-time friends actresses Vicki and Annie Michelle, who encouraged me to be very positive in my attitude. I've felt pretty wet up until now and

I really must get a grip – I know I'll feel better once I've transferred to the Marsden and had my ultrasound.

FRIDAY 15TH JUNE:
Tears Before Bedtime

I had an appointment with the surgeon at the Charing Cross. I was still feeling pretty sorry for myself but, as I walked in, I saw a woman sitting outside the hospital in a wheelchair. As I got closer I realised the poor lady had no legs. It really put things into perspective – you can easily get around with one less breast, but your legs... I felt very humble.

At my appointment, the surgeon asked me what Mr Gui had said and got very cross when I said he was hoping to do a wide local excision only. She said she refused to do 'that operation' on me and that I wouldn't get a good result either health-wise or aesthetically – but she couldn't explain why not. She then said she could refer me to other surgeons at the hospital who *would* do the operation I wanted. I was really confused – who were these surgeons and were they more skilled or less skilled than this one? Anyway, Mr Gui was legendary; I certainly didn't need any other surgeons to do the smaller operation.

I tentatively asked to see some pictures of some of her former patients who had had the mastectomy operation she was planning to do on me. When she showed me, I burst into tears. Those poor women, what must they have suffered? The operations looked so cruel and painful, with such huge scars. Was a mastectomy really a healthier option?

Aesthetically, the operated breasts looked completely different from the healthy ones, rock solid and six inches higher. I could understand why MX – that's the short name for mastectomy – patients often later opted to have the healthy breast operated on to match the 'done' one.

Then the surgeon said I would have to have a fake nipple put on at a later stage as well – cue for fresh waterworks! I would be having operations at this hospital for months if I wanted my boobs to look OK for evening dress endorsements!

Nurse Addie wasn't there and the surgeon was frantically ringing her – to calm me down, I guess. (Later on, I realised that the two times I had been treated less than kindly at the Charing Cross Hospital breast unit was when there had been no nice breast nurse there as a buffer.)

ADVICE: *If you feel you are being bullied or patronised by a surgeon, ask to have a nurse there – it's your right as a vulnerable cancer patient. I imagine cancer care nurses are chosen for their kind nature and maybe Addie would have understood my pain and could have explained what I needed to know.*

In any case, my ten minutes was up and I stumbled out of the room. As I left, the surgeon put her hand on my shoulder and said: 'Be strong. Take my strength', and I thought 'Oh, she's not so bad after all' but then I realised that there were people standing outside the door who would see how upset I was.

I went into the loo and cried my heart out: a very dark day. At least now I wouldn't feel guilty about transferring my care from one hospital to the other any more and I later got onto my GP's surgery about it.

ADVICE: Not everybody knows that you can transfer your NHS care from one hospital to another. This is really valuable information. I later spoke to an old friend who said her oncologist had been consistently unkind to her and this is simply not on with any patient, let alone a vulnerable cancer patient. Doctors owe you a duty of care – it's the Hippocratic oath, not the hypocritical oath! You can change your specialist and you can change your hospital.

Later I took Jade to Harvey Nichols' sale to get her a dress for Ascot and found a gorgeous purple Pucci number. I also found a cheapo pink evening dress for myself – retail therapy is most uplifting (excuse the pun!). You couldn't wear a bra with this dress so this was a real act of defiance for me – I must trust that I will only need the smaller operation.

That evening I went to see my lawyer friend Michael Cooper. Both he and his nephew who was there were extremely kind to me and said that guys don't really care about specific bits of our female bods, it's the whole package that counts and that, even if I *did* eventually have to have a MX, I would still have my face and my legs... I feel really sorry for ladies who have fantastic boobs (I don't, mine are just ordinary) and have to sacrifice one. MX is such a big one, for the psyche as well as the health.

MONDAY 18TH JUNE:
First Ultrasound

I had my ultrasound at the Marsden. I only had to wait a short time and then a nice radiologist called Nancy did the test, which was like the ultrasounds I'd had when pregnant, and completely painless. The good news is that some little lumps in my armpits are completely benign. Nancy then showed me my tumour on the screen; it looked like two small lumps but she said it could be two halves of the same lump. Anyway, it didn't look very big and it hasn't spread into the lymph nodes, so I was totally elated!

Nancy also told me that nowadays there are no surprises with breast surgery: they won't take out more tissue than they say they will. Apparently in the old days patients would go to sleep not knowing what the surgeons would find in there and not knowing if they would wake up having had a lumpectomy or a mastectomy. OMG, terrible! We are so lucky to live in this modern generation.

ADVICE: Everybody says that breast cancer is one of the 'best' cancers, because it is very treatable if diagnosed early. Ask your doctor to teach you how to examine your breasts yourself if you don't want to have a mammogram because of the radiation.

WEDNESDAY 20TH JUNE:
The Professor Explains Chemotherapy

I went to the Marsden General Outpatients Department to see the famous Professor Smith and his oncology team. There is a nice little café there and a bookstand. I bought three books and the tactful café lady said she thought I would do well with my treatment as I looked very fit in my cycling pants – well, I think everyone looks fit in cycling pants!

As I opened one of the books, out fell a ticket from the Royal Academy of Arts with a lady's name printed on it. I wondered if that lady had been a patient, if she had survived, how she was now... Everything is making me cry at the moment. Is it normal or am I just a super wimp?

I then saw Geraldine, Professor Smith's secretary, Andreas, his registrar, senior staff nurse, Elena, and the Professor himself. They were all so nice and friendly and I was so glad that I am officially registered at the Marvellous Marsden. My hospital number is 603561.

Professor Smith is a delightful, slim, silver-haired chap and his mellifluous Dundee tones soothed my nerves. He explained they were thinking of giving me chemo first, before surgery, to shrink the lump and make it more easily operable. Chemo would also 'mop up' any microscopic bad cells floating around. He wanted to do a Ki67 tumour marker test to determine how quickly the tumour might be spreading and if it would respond to chemo. At more or less 3 centimetres, mine is apparently considered large for a lump. I can feel it myself now I know where it is but as I've said before, the doctors discourage you from feeling your lumps as it may inflame them.

The Professor said I would have the chemo intravenously (ouch!) – two drugs called 'EC' (Epirubicin and Cyclophosphamide) first, every three weeks x four times, followed by a drug called 'Taxol' every two weeks x four times, making five months of chemo in all. The tumour would be monitored with ultrasound after every two cycles and, if it didn't respond to the EC, they would switch to the Taxol more quickly.

He then ran through all the side-effects while I tried to keep my fixed smile in place: hair loss, maybe lash and brow loss, skin dryness, tingling of fingertips, infections (although these were not usually life-threatening), tiredness... But he also said that nowadays they had medication to control the vomiting and nausea, thank God.

I asked about having scalp cooling to prevent hair loss and he said that it's not really painful and often worked, though not always.

The Prof said he'd treated lots of actresses and models before and that they'd usually done very well and been able to work quite a lot. Maybe the old stage 'trouper' mentality would help me. At any rate he is very reassuring and inspiring and I was so glad Tatiana had suggested him to me – it was literally a lifesaver! The Prof also generously offered to check my book for medical accuracy, which is a huge boon – I can't even pronounce the names of the chemo treatments I'm going to have!

THURSDAY 21ST JUNE:
Ladies' Day At Royal Ascot

Jeremy and I took Jade – resplendent in her Pucci frock – and Allie, and met up with Charlotte, Nora Seroussi and various other friends at that fabulous social event, Royal Ascot. My pal Suzanne had bagged a great table in our favourite seafood restaurant and, awash with champagne, I soon forgot my health woes. One of my doctors had told me that champagne is good for my spirits at the moment – actually, I think it's good for me all the time! Poncing about in the Royal Enclosure in a huge hat, chatting to friends and losing money on the geegees, I felt very jolly and not at all like a person who was about to start cancer treatment.

FRIDAY 22ND JUNE:
The Price Of Saving Your Life

My photographer friend Rowena Chowdrey met me for tea at the Hurlingham Club. She was photographing a tournament there and I was spectating. She told me she had had two friends who had had breast cancer. One had gone privately and it had cost her £40,000 but she had survived. The other had tragically died after being misdiagnosed at her local hospital and therefore treated too late. Awful.

I believe the total private cost of breast cancer treatment, including surgery, chemo, radio and medication now stands at £50,000. It's a huge sum for most people to find, but who can put a value on your life?

SATURDAY 23RD JUNE:
Advice From Cancer Survivors

I saw my friend the fashion designer Charles Svingholm who had recently been through chemotherapy for Hodgkin's lymphoma. I knew that he had been extremely ill and that it had badly affected his normally thriving business but, thank goodness, he was now completely better.

Charlie told me I would feel extremely tired with chemo and that I absolutely must <u>not</u> catch any infections or I would have to be hospitalised, as he had been, in isolation, on various occasions. That sounded awful, but I knew he'd had chemo on a weekly, rather than a three-weekly basis, and mine being more spread out would give me a chance to recover before each successive round.

Charlie confirmed many of the side-effects the Prof had told me about. He was the only person I'd talked to who said his hair had *not* grown back thicker and curlier than before – but maybe that was because he is a guy? Certainly his lashes look divine now – thick, curly and totally envy-making. He also said that you can get terrible constipation from chemo. I remember some poor film star in the newspapers who had had to get her boyfriend to dig her 'faecal matter' out with a spoon! That is so not going to happen to me, I vowed, as I mentally stocked up on Bran Flakes and prune juice.

'Then there is the insomnia all the time,' he said, which plunged me into further gloom as I suffer from mild insomnia already.

Later on I spoke to a lady called Ann, who my mate Vicki Michelle had put me in touch with. Ann had sadly lost her mum to breast cancer but survived herself after having an initial lumpectomy followed by a third of her breast removed some years ago. She sounded very cheerful and upbeat and I admired her spirit. Ann told me that the DCIS mentioned on my histology was actually Ductal Carcinoma In Situ and we worked out between us that, if it was 'in situ' in the ducts, it wasn't going anywhere, i.e. spreading – and this was brilliant news!

ADVICE: Talk to people who have been through it before; this is so valuable.

Even if you have the best doctors in the business – and I know now that I have, thank goodness – it's always good to speak to women who have actually had breast cancer, and men and women who have been through chemo. Fear of the unknown is very stressful and it's reassuring to know what to expect. Each case is different and unique but I am learning so much by talking to friends and friends of friends. One of my cousins has also written to me to say he'd survived cancer – he's young, the poor thing, and I'd never known. In this book I thank all of those people for the precious time they so generously gave me when they told me their stories and discussed them with me.

SUNDAY 24TH JUNE:
Advice Before Chemo

A long time friend of mine, Gloria Stuart, had put me in touch with a very friendly and upbeat cancer survivor called Marianne. She gave me the following excellent advice via email: *'Cut out all dairy products to ward off nausea, use aloe vera on the skin following radiotherapy, get a soft little baby's hat to wear on your head if you go bald, and sort out a good wig in advance of any hair loss.'*

Marianne also told me that, if I *did* have to have a mastectomy, the reconstruction of the nipple bit was painless due to local anaesthetic. I'd always felt particularly squeamish about that bit.

I'd got used to cutting out dairy when the Harley Street

doctor had put me on a no wheat/no dairy regime after my bad laryngitis last year, which was just as well as I hate feeling nauseous. Vomiting is anathema to me – I could never be bulimic!

Marianne also said that Mr Gui had done an amazing reconstruction on a friend of hers. I am feeling so much more confident now that I am in such good hands.

I received another lovely – and philosophical – email from my friend Margaret from 'oop North' who wrote: '*I just know karma couldn't let anything happen to a good person like you and you will get through it OK. I'm not saying it will be easy, but life's not easy.*' I've never thought of myself as a particularly good person before but I truly believe that going through cancer and seeing others suffer around you definitely makes you a better person: more humble, compassionate and grateful.

TUESDAY 26TH JUNE:
Advice Before Chemo

David Goodman, a friend who has a reputation as an amazing healer, came round to work on me. I had written out a potted medical history for him. He said that my cancer had not come from within me but from something traumatic that had happened to me six years ago. I was fairly sure I knew what that was – but that's another book!

David's treatment included the laying-on of hands and deep breathing (him, not me) and made me feel totally relaxed – I almost fell asleep. I hope it helps – I certainly felt good afterwards.

WEDNESDAY 27TH JUNE:
Consultation Re Breast Conserving Surgery

To the Marsden to see Mr Gui again to discuss 'breast conservation surgery' further. Regarding the size of my lump, Mr Gui said that, although 3 centimetres sounds small, when you considered the margin that he would have to take out around it as well and the relatively small size of the breast (I am only a C cup in my padded bra!), it was not so small. I believe 3 centimetres is considered quite a 'big' lump and only 2 centimetres and below are considered 'small'.

He said the results of the Ki67 test would determine if I had chemo before surgery or not. The course of chemo would be around five months or so, with three weeks in between before surgery, and then three to four weeks of radiotherapy afterwards. I was looking at being 'off games', as we'd say at school, for around nine to ten months. Then we discussed scalp cooling with chemo – I definitely want it, even if it is really uncomfortable.

I also had a long chat with Vanda, another very helpful breast nurse. She gave me a booklet on breast reconstruction, with lots of pictures of reconstructions. These didn't look nearly as scary as the ones the surgeon from the Charing Cross had shown me but I still appreciated what a big operation a MX is, involving a few days in hospital. I know from talking to various people that some patients still have to have a MX at a later stage after a lumpectomy but I feel very strongly that I should try the minor surgery first.

There were no pictures of lumpectomies in the booklet –

maybe because the results are so much less visible – well, I'm hoping mine will be anyway! Vanda felt my back and said there was no flesh there for the reconstruction: 'You're so thin!' she said. I realise that being a skinny-minny I am not an ideal patient aesthetically for reconstruction but health-wise I will have whatever is necessary.

That evening I drank red wine for the first time and quite liked it. Everybody, especially my cancer knowledgeable friend and house guest Adele, says red wine is actually good for you and that I must swap white for red. Jeremy found me a light fruity red, which you drink chilled, at the local Tesco and I decided I could quite get into it.

FRIDAY 29TH JUNE:
Mastectomy Without Reconstruction

To the Hurlingham Club for Victoria, Ian and Lucinda Watson's fun 'Heroes And Villains' party, co-organised by Victoria's event organiser sister, Liz Brewer, so it was excellent. I went as the Wicked Queen wearing one of Jade's fancy dress frocks, which had great big Madonna-type cones on the boobs (I wonder how much longer I will get away with drawing attention to them?) and had a great time.

My friend Cindy Jackson, the cosmetic surgery guru, was wearing an amazing wig and said she would give me her 'wiggly' contacts if necessary.

Sitting next to me was a charming older lady who kept adjusting her jacket. I could see that she had some uncomfortable-looking padding and had clearly had a mastectomy and wondered if she would talk to me about it. I broke the ice by mentioning my situation and she opened up to me. She said she had also been under the care of Professor Smith and Mr Gui at the Marsden and had had the operation successfully with no recurrence of the cancer.

She seemed to be an incredibly brave and down-to-earth lady who had had her operation brought forward so that she could still go off on a planned holiday! She hadn't wanted a reconstruction and had just got on with her busy life with her business, her children and grandchildren. I so much admired her for choosing not to reconstruct, with all the attendant time, trouble and discomfort, but hoped that she would find a more comfortable bra and padding – maybe one of those nice soft gel jobbies.

SATURDAY 30TH JUNE:
Getting It Off My Chest!

Charlotte, my PR and good friend, had very cleverly booked me to do an article for the Daily Mail, who were publishing quite a lot about mastectomies at the time, and it appeared today. The Mail's agenda was to find someone who wanted a lumpectomy instead of a MX for aesthetic reasons and the editing and headline reflected the aesthetic over the health issues. However, I got my message out there that surgeons shouldn't be too quick to whip off the whole breast if the minor lumpectomy operation would be just as successful, health-wise and aesthetically, for the patient.

I realise that I may be left with a dent in my breast after the lumpectomy but I don't actually care because it's on the outside of the boob, which doesn't show in dresses and I will still have my cleavage which is the bit of the bustline I need for my work. Health-wise, if I can have a minor rather than a major operation just as safely for the cancer, I must do that. If I have to have chemo and radio anyway, the less time spent on surgery and reconstruction the better.

I got a very good response to the article – which sported glamorous pictures by the talented Brian Aris – via the paper, online, from friends and from people I didn't know. Some had been through what I'd been through at the Charing Cross, probably with the same doctors. All were very supportive of my fight for women not to be bullied into a MX if they only need a lumpectomy.

Today was my God-daughter Isabella Bruce's wedding to her fiancé (now husband) Ben, and I had a lovely time at the wedding with Jade and Jeremy, and Bella's parents Johnny and Erica, who are Godparents to Jade. It was so nice to get away from thoughts of hospitals, treatments and cancer for a while and watch Bella waft up the aisle in her gorgeous white dress looking like an angel! I thoroughly recommend carrying on an active social life if you can, to take your mind off your illness.

SUNDAY 1ST JULY:
A Journey And The Journey

Carrying on my taking-your-mind-off-it social life, I went down to see some fun friends in the West Country, where Andrew Rogers was holding his birthday dinner party at Sir Benjamin Slade's stunning country estate. My friend Princess Katarina kindly drove. Andrew and Benjy were on cracking form and my old friend Alexander Bath (the famous Marquess!) was also there with his regular 'wifelet,' Trudie. The party was amazing and I met all sorts of interesting new folks. Andrew had kindly got in lots of soy milk and fresh fruit for me and I really enjoyed sleeping in the four-poster in the Lady Slade room and eating cooked breakfast and porridge the next day. Benjy's nice PA, Naomi, gave me an inspirational book about cancer healing called *The Journey*, by Brandon Bays, a lady who got rid of her tumour through healing and diet alone. I can't wait to read it.

WEDNESDAY 4TH JULY:
Results Of The Ki67 Test

Off to the Marsden again with Jade. Professor Smith was away so I saw Dr Turner. He is head of a research programme and I signed some forms for two research programmes I've agreed to participate in.

Dr Turner said they'd finally got the results of the Ki67 test (the Charing Cross Breast Unit had initially sent the wrong tissue samples so there had been a hold-up.) He said mine was an aggressive, faster-growing cancer and that it would definitely benefit from chemo; I could expect shrinkage of the tumour and that chemo would increase the cure and kill off any breast cancer I had. He reiterated that I would have to have chemo whether I had a MX or lumpectomy and that I should start the course in a week or two (help!) We then discussed the chemo treatment and side-effects again. Dr Turner told me to get a thermometer and take my temperature regularly if I felt at all feverish. If my temperature went above 38 degrees I would have to be hospitalised for safety.

Like most ladies, I was worried about potential hair loss and the doctor said I should start the scalp cooling forty-five minutes before the actual chemo treatment. He also said I would not be able to colour my hair during the cancer course. That's fine because my hair is quite blonde anyway and I only usually need a few highlights. However I was worried that, if I lost my hair at my age it might grow back grey, as had happened with other people I know.

I also discussed HRT. At the suggestion of Mr Gui's team I had gone off HRT after being on it for a few years and my hormonal symptoms had returned, plus I was feeling more tired and stressed than usual. However, that could be due to my natural worry about my disease and fear of the treatment and Dr Turner suggested that, now I was off HRT I should stay off it. I didn't know it at that stage but there were much worse things than tiredness and stress ahead of me!

Then I bumped into senior staff nurse Elena who said that chemo was actually an excellent treatment and she was pleased I would be having it and that the doctors thought it would work well on me. She warned me that, if the cancer returned, I would have to have a second round of chemo. This news made me all the more determined to stick to the Cancer Diet and my complementary treatments if I can, to ward off a return of the cancer. Elena said that chemo had been given to pregnant ladies with no harmful effects to mother and baby and that many ladies who had chemo went on to have healthy pregnancies. I guess that's a pretty good sign that chemo is not the awful killer many people say it is. To a mother there is nothing more precious in your body than a baby.

Next I had to have a blood test to make sure my white cell count was high enough to tolerate chemo. My blood was taken by Freddie from Ghana, a very jolly gentleman I later named 'Freddie The Blood'! With the sympathetic Freddie it was only a little scratch and I averted my eyes from the actual bottles of blood – I'm so blood and needle phobic.

As I retrieved my car, Violet, I decided to inspect the attractive restaurant opposite the Marsden, Le Columbier, as I'd worked out that I would be spending a lot of time at the hospital and that the restaurant might be a good new HQ for me. As things worked out, I was not in the end up to eating much rich food whilst being treated for cancer!

THURSDAY 5TH JULY:
Introduction To 'Cancer Options'

A 'bionic woman' friend – the inspiring Janie Martel – had also been treated at the Marsden by Professor Smith, whom she admired greatly. Janie suggested that to answer all the questions I might forget to ask at the hospital, I also consult Patricia Peat from Cancer Options, via Yes To Life. This is a charity run by Robin Daly, which I was now supporting along with Janie. One of the wonderful things that Yes To Life – which is staffed totally by volunteers – does is to sponsor consultations with Patricia, a respected former oncology nurse who now runs Cancer Options. She helps people with cancer make informed choices and put them in charge of their own cancer treatment, and the charity had now kindly agreed to sponsor me. Janie had told me that Patricia was absolutely brilliant and I was most impressed with her patience, kindness and thoroughness in the phone consultation I had with her.

Patricia later sent me her advice from my consultation – a huge dossier with invaluable information that I refer to regularly. The most important questions for me at the time were:

'Will chemo kill any cancer anywhere in my body?' YES!

'Does chemo shorten your life?' NO!

'If I have it before surgery, will I also need it afterwards?' Probably not.

'Might chemo shrink the tumour away completely?' It's possible.

'If the breast cancer has not spread to the lymph glands, will it not have spread further?' Usually not.

I mentioned my friend Georgina, who had survived breast cancer and then sadly died of ovarian cancer a few years later, and Patricia said that was very unusual and she might have had something called 'Brecker's Disease' which one is unlikely to get if it is not in the family.

We also discussed the ticklish problem of hair loss. Patricia said it usually occurred after the second session of chemo and that it would probably fall out from all over the head with no scalp cooling and from different areas of the head even if I *did* have the cooling – which I understand is *extremely* cool. Patricia confirmed what my doctors and nutritionist had told me: that I should be as fit as possible before starting chemo. I knew that I wasn't, due to the state of my immune system, so all I could do was stick to the Cancer Diet – which I was beginning to find easier – keep exercising, and pray!

FRIDAY 6TH JULY:
Breast Cancer Survivor Nicky's Story

One of my husband Jeremy's best friends is also called Jeremy (Mitchell) and his wife Nicky had had breast cancer eight years ago. Nicky rang me today and told me that she had had exactly what I was to have and it had been completely successful, with no recurrence after eight years! So reassuring. She had sensibly had health insurance, so had been treated at our local private hospital, The Cromwell. The whole treatment, including lumpectomy surgery, chemo, radio and medication (five years of Tamoxifen) had totted up to between £40,000 and £50,000! (I am *so* glad I am being treated so well at the Marsden on the NHS, so lucky.)

Nicky said that she felt woozy after chemo and that I would need a 'chemo buddy' to take me home afterwards; it also made her feel nauseous. She said that she ditched the 'ice cap' because it was so cold and uncomfortable and yes, her hair did fall out, though she didn't bother to shave it, and her brows and lashes too, but they all grew back again. She warned that the first three days after chemo are pretty grim but you gradually get better and better over the next two-and-a-half weeks – then you have to have it all over again! Nicky said that she didn't try to do much while on chemo, just rested, watched telly, read and occasionally took the dogs for a walk. She lost her appetite but developed a craving for houmous and avocados.

She did say that, because the chemo treatment involves steroids (to counteract the nausea) she put on weight and her face would swell up at the beginning of the cycle. I have to remember this was eight years ago and I feel sure they have made vast improvements, as the researchers and medics are finessing cancer treatments all the time.

Nicky's lump was 2 to 3 centimetres, like mine, but the cancer was already Stage 3 and it had spread to her lymph glands, so those had to be removed too. Her surgery went well and she then had radiotherapy for six weeks. She said she got accumulated tiredness from radiotherapy and also reddened skin, though this was soothed with aloe vera (also recommended by Marianne).

She warned me to stay out of the sun after radiotherapy, which made me wonder when Jade and I would achieve our dream of going to Atlantis, the beautiful hotel on Paradise Island in the Bahamas, to frolic with the dolphins!

One of the things Nicky mentioned was that her lump had *not* shown up on a mammogram and that she always has ultrasound scans now. The really good news was that she went back to normal within a week or so after chemo, which certainly seems to be the worst time during cancer treatment. The very best news is that eight years later she is completely cancer free.

SATURDAY 7TH JULY:
Cancer Tragedies

I tottered up to Maida Vale to visit my old friend, actor and national treasure Leslie Phillips. Leslie went through a terrible time after his actress wife Angela Scoular survived a year of ovarian cancer, whipped it – and then committed suicide. An appalling tragedy.

Just recently Leslie had also lost one of his best friends, Robin Gibb, to cancer. Robin had bravely gone off on a world tour with the Bee Gees knowing that it would probably be his last but not wanting to let the band down. Another dreadful tragedy. His poor family – and poor Leslie. However, Leslie had one bit of good news and showed me a card from a lady friend who had just had the all clear after having breast cancer. I promised him I intended to beat it myself and he was very impressed that I was already on the Cancer Diet, drinking green tea and refusing my usual cakes and biscuits!

SUNDAY 8TH JULY:
Pre–MRI Scan

I was given a surprise birthday party, kindly hosted by Jeremy, at Da Mario on Queensgate Terrace, my old HQ when I'd lived a few doors up for several years. It wasn't my exact birthday but what the hell! It cheered me up no end to see all my mates and have pasta and wine (red, now that I'm on the famous Cancer Diet!)

I was going for an MRI (Magnetic Resonance Imaging)

scan the next day to get a closer look at my tumour and my pals Vivien and Steven said I would need to take a Valium before it. I had been told it wasn't painful but immediately texted the doctor who replied that it 'wasn't scary, no pain' so I wouldn't need the Valium. Goodo, I could have more to drink!

MONDAY 9TH JULY:
MRI Scan

I went to Guy's Hospital at London Bridge for the MRI as they had some new and exciting technology whereby they could later do an ultrasound whilst looking at MRI results to get really up close and personal with my lump.

The MRI staff were all adorable but I was devastated to discover that I had to have an injection and they would pass a dye through my vein and that I would be able to feel the liquid coursing up the vein. This is my worst nightmare after a dreadful experience I had with an anaesthetic for an emergency operation, when the anaesthetist had put the drug in quickly and I had felt like a criminal being executed by lethal injection!

So during the blooming MRI I was sobbing but trying not to heave, as you have to lie completely still with your head and each boob in a hole for the tests, which took around twenty minutes in all. I had been warned about the loud clanking noise that accompanied the MRI and had taken the suggested calming music to play in my headphones. However I couldn't hear the music at all and recommend to MRI patients that you wear earplugs instead – just like HM The Queen at the Diamond Jubilee Concert in her own back yard!

ADVICE: MRI SCANS. I was a nervous wreck when I came out and suggest that all patients of a nervous disposition or who, like me, are needle-phobic, do indeed take a Lorazepam (an anti-anxiety pill) before the test if having the injection as well. The test itself, without the injection, isn't too bad, just noisy – but you need to take a friend or family member to take you home afterwards if taking a Lorazepam.

Naturally I had to have a large drink when I got home and was very disappointed that the doctor had clearly bamboozled me. He later said: 'If we told patients what it was like, they wouldn't have it'. I think that is totally underestimating the courage and determination of cancer patients. We just want to get better.

ADVICE: Always check exactly what each test involves and Be Prepared, as the Boy Scouts say! There is no shame in taking a pill if you are scared and friends and family are usually happy to be involved and accompany you to any test or treatment where you need support. Ask your medical team to always tell you the truth; you need to trust your doctors. Stress from pain and anxiety should be kept to a minimum as it exacerbates cancer.

TUESDAY 10TH JULY:
PICC Lines, Wig Consultation And Hypnotherapy

Back to the Marsden with Jade again, where nurse Melanie kindly and patiently talked me through the chemo process again, assuring me I would get the best anti-nausea drug, Ondemet, to take home with me as well as having the steroids they give you with the EC chemo drugs. She also said I would have a heated blanket to keep me warm while having the 'ice cap', which is what scalp cooling is.

I felt sick as a dog with fear before even starting the treatment; just the word 'chemotherapy' turned my blood to ice. It was mainly fear of the unknown, not knowing how painful it would be and if I would let myself down and cry when they put those huge cannulas into my delicate feminine little veins! Would there be blood? Would I faint? Oh God, oh God, oh God – I began to think I should not take Jade with me the first time as I did not want her to be upset if it was really awful.

Melanie advised me to keep up my exercise regime if I could but said I would feel pretty tired throughout the chemo course. She said that the younger and fitter you are, the less tired you will feel. They consider a patient of my (middle) age 'young' by cancer standards. I must say I was feeling ancient just hearing about the treatment – I am such a wuss!

Then I met Yukie, the clinical research nurse for one of the research programmes I had agreed to. She was adorable, like a little Japanese doll. She explained that I would have various core biopsies, ultrasounds and blood tests throughout my chemo treatment to monitor how the tumour reacted to it.

I trembled at the thought of all these extra needles but senior staff nurse Elena later told me if necessary I could have a permanent PICC line (peripherally inserted central catheter) put in which stays in my vein throughout and through which *all* the IVs could be given to me.

ADVICE: Instead of a permanent PICC line (which sounds very serious and may be more suitable for those poor patients who are in and out of hospital on a regular basis), Elena advised me to request a Lorazepam and anaesthetic gel on the skin over my vein half an hour before chemo.

All this talk of needles was making me edgy so Jade and I went over the road to Le Columbier for a glass of champagne (recommended by one of my doctors!) and delicious fish soup, after which I felt much better.

My next stop was at the Marsden hairdressing department to choose a wig in advance of hair loss, as Marianne had suggested. When we walked in, Paul the friendly wig master said: 'Which of you ladies is it for?' and both Jade and I were very sad to think that girls as young as her could be suffering from cancer. But sadly I know it's true, having seen a beautiful young black girl in Outpatients recently with a huge hat on, presumably going through chemo. I determined to encourage both Jade and my 'step-in' daughter Kat, whose poor mum Marilyn had also had breast cancer, you may remember, to check themselves regularly while they are still considered too young to get a reliable mammogram test (because the breast tissue is apparently too dense in young women).

Paul found me a lovely long blonde, slightly Dolly Parton type wiggly called 'Crystal' by Natural Image and ordered it for me in two different colours to try. He explained that the ice cap doesn't necessarily prevent the hair falling out, just prolongs it – and if your hair becomes too thin with too many bald patches, you will not be able to continue with the cap because you will get frostbite!

Later that afternoon, hypnotherapist Lucien Morgan came round to work his magic on me and calm me down before my round of intravenous injections and to work on my feelings about needles and blood. 'Luce' gave me two different types of hypnotherapy to regress me to the situations that gave me the phobias, and to forget them. He then taught me self hypnosis, which will be extremely valuable for putting myself into a 'trance' for each round of chemo, core biopsies or anything else that frightens me and to help fight the insomnia I am likely to get with chemo.

He said I was a great patient for hypno. I'd previously been treated successfully for 'choo choo phobia' (fear of trains!), smoking and insomnia by Lucien's colleague Valerie Austin, so I was already a huge fan of hypno and immediately felt more confident about all the treatments after just one session with Lucien.

WEDNESDAY 11TH JULY:
Keep Socialising!

I was on the committee for the Conservative Party's Two Cities Lunch organised by Paddy Evershed (chairman of the Cities of London and Westminster Conservative Association) with speakers William Hague and our MP, Mark Field. I took my pal and cancer supporter Ruth along to join Peter Stringfellow, who was kindly hosting a table. Good company, food and wine and excellent speeches took my mind off illness. Ruth is really helpful, having supported 'bionic' Janie through not just breast cancer but many of her health problems. It was also great to sit next to Peter, a very kind and generous person as well as a national treasure, who was on his usual ebullient form.

I'd first met Peter in 1980 when he opened Stringfellow's with a fabulous launch party. I was working at the Arts Theatre across the road doing my first West End leading role in Sir Tom Stoppard's *Dirty Linen* but was only a young and relatively unknown actress, so didn't get an invite. However, our leading man, the famous Peter Bowles, was invited and he kindly got me in. I became firm friends with Stringfellows and its owner and have had some wonderful evenings and parties there and at Peter's other club, Angels, ever since. Peter and Ruth and co cheered me up no end and took my mind off the terror of my impending treatment.

THURSDAY 12TH JULY:
Two Lumps, Not One

Back to Guy's to have the new ultrasound, where they could view my MRI results at the same time. The lovely ladies in the imaging suite all crowded round me to check out the cutting-edge new technology – and it was fascinating. I could clearly see on the screen that I had not one but two lumps, one tiny and one bigger but totalling in all just under 3 centimetres. Now I know exactly what we are dealing with and I'm so glad I'd had the MRI. The radiologist also found a small lump under my arm which she biopsied but it was later found to be benign, thank goodness.

FRIDAY 13TH JULY:
Procrastination And The Journey

Jade and I drove down to Longleat, the Marquess of Bath's beautiful ancestral home, to discuss possibly holding Jade's upcoming 21st birthday party there. It was Friday 13th, lashing down with rain, and I got lost – I don't usually drive myself to Longleat. I was really calm about it all and realised that Lucien's hypnotherapy had already done me a power of good in under twenty-four hours. After looking around the possible rooms where we could throw this great bash, we popped up to Alexander's penthouse apartment to visit him and his doggies and were pleased to find him on great form. Now if only I can be on great form for Jade's birthday: I will have to work out my chemo dates and my 'good' periods.

I was getting one of my usual colds and asked Geraldine, Professor Smith's super-efficient secretary, if I could put off my chemo from next Monday 'til later in the week. I so want to be super-fit when I start the dreaded chemo but it doesn't look like I am going to be. Since being diagnosed with cancer, I have tried really hard to eat lots of fresh fruit and veg, organic and good stuff, ditch the microwave and the TV dinners but the jolly old British summer weather isn't helping me to get over my cold!

At home that night I finished reading Brandon Bays' wonderful book, *The Journey*. She really deserved to cure her tumour naturally, living on a diet of fresh fruit and veg only for weeks on end and, being a healer, working on herself. I knew I could never achieve that myself but was keen to eat as well as I could and carry on with David

Goodman's excellent healing as a complement to the orthodox medical route I was taking.

Brandon Bays is an inspiring woman. She says: 'When life gives you lemons, make lemonade'. Well, I think I might have said 'Frozen Margaritas' but I know I need to cut down on alcohol if I really, really want to whip cancer!

Brandon Bays also said that all she really needed in life was to earn enough money to 'put food in our bellies' and we can all relate to that.

ADVICE: As we get older, we are all likely to need more health maintenance and if, like foolish me, you don't have health insurance and a job that compensates you if you're ill, you should put some money aside. The NHS will take care of your medical needs but you still need money to live and don't need the pressure of having to get back to earning a living asap.

SATURDAY 14TH JULY:
Intraoperative Radiation Therapy – And In Memory of Bryony

I had a further chat with Patricia Peat from Cancer Options. I had heard about a new operation for breast cancer called 'intraoperative radiation therapy', where they give you a big targeted dose of radiotherapy at the time of removing the tumour, rather than having to go through up to six weeks of tiring radiotherapy after surgery. This would help me get back to work, 'putting food in our bellies' more quickly after surgery, and Patricia advised me to go for it if I could. 'Be a health tourist, look around for all your possible options,' she said. I told her that my lumps were sore at the moment and she said that it was quite natural for them to be inflamed after all the tests.

Patricia said that recovery after cancer is really down to the individual and I should keep up my complementary treatments as well as going the orthodox route. She also told me the sad story of why Robin Daly had started the Yes To Life charity. His daughter Bryony had had cancer as a child and had recovered but had then suffered bone cancer caused by excessive radiotherapy, which could not be treated. Tragically she had died in her early twenties and they hadn't found out about alternative treatments until too late. Robin started the charity to help others. I am so glad that I am now supporting Yes To Life. Losing your child is the worst thing that can happen to any parent and I so admire Robin.

SUNDAY 15TH JULY:
A Hospital Tragedy

The hospital where my friend Anna worked, St George's in Tooting, south west London, was in the news for the wrong reason. A young patient had died after becoming dehydrated. Apparently the staff were all extremely busy, hadn't read his notes and didn't give him his special medication, so he became aggressive – whereupon they sedated him and were then too busy to give him a drink of water. He died in his mother's arms at the hospital. A terrible tragedy and a sad lesson to us all.

I am determined not to be hospitalised if I can possibly help it. A lumpectomy should be a day job and I must avoid catching infections like my poor friend Charlie, who had to be hospitalised regularly.

MONDAY 16TH JULY:
Alternatives To Chemo?

I had a long talk with 'bionic woman' Janie Martel, who was horrified that I was going the chemo route. She said that the Germans and Swiss were so far ahead of us in treating cancer and that she had had a treatment at a German clinic where they just use chemo on the actual tumour, not the whole body. Apparently it costs about £20,000 but if you have the money, go for it! Janie had actually been extremely ill in many ways and unable to tolerate traditional British chemo, so it worked for her.

I am just a normal person and not otherwise ill, so I should be able to tolerate traditional chemo. However I did think about it and even considered paying $3,000 to a Harley Street doctor who could send my tissue samples to Switzerland – or was it America – to be analysed, so I'd know for sure if I needed chemo or not. However it would take two to three weeks and I didn't really have the time any more.

My friend Christine, who had bowel cancer (later operated on successfully), told me about a clinic in Dallas where they guaranteed a cancer cure for everybody, even people who had been given six weeks to live! Good to investigate if you or a loved one are terminal...

I was not that ill but I realised I must get on with it. Things came to the crunch later that evening when Jade and I were watching *Britain's Next Top Model* and one of the girls had a tattoo for her mum who had died from breast cancer. Looking at my daughter's stricken face I knew that on Wednesday, when I had another meeting with the doctors at the Marsden, I had to make a decision once and for all.

TUESDAY 17TH JULY:
Fresh Air And Exercise

I played tennis with my three 'J' boys, James, James and Jeremy, at Hurlingham and wondered if I would be well enough to play the following week. Afterwards I drank water instead of wine or coffee but treated myself to some peanuts – a big thrill!

WEDNESDAY 18TH JULY:
Pre-Chemo Fears

In Mr Gui's absence I saw Mrs Agusti on the surgical breast team at the Marsden. I would really have preferred to have had surgery first but both she and my breast nurse Melanie agreed that I should have chemo first to try to shrink the tumour, which was what my oncologist Professor Smith thought was best. They said that if the tumour hadn't shrunk after two cycles of EC chemo they would change the treatment or maybe have surgery earlier. Of course if the tumour *did* shrink it would mean a smaller dent in the breast, although Mrs Agusti did say that they would pull the tissues together to fill it up and I could always have a fat transfer three weeks after the end of my chemo and radio treatments (or six weeks after if they had to remove any lymph as well as breast tissue.) They guaranteed that the tumour absolutely would *not* grow during chemo.

As I looked into Mrs Agusti and Mel's kind concerned faces, I was shaking with fear and once more felt physically sick at the thought of starting chemotherapy. How could I get out of it? Could I put it off again? Then I thought of Jade's little face and realised I couldn't put her, my innocent young daughter, through any more anxiety and distress. I bit the bullet and agreed to sign the chemo consent form the following day and have my first session on Friday.

Of course, I was still worried about possible hair loss and had a long chat with trichologist Richard Spencer from The Spencer Clinic. He said that if I did lose my hair it would grow back again at the rate of about 1 centimetre per month but that I could have treatment to stimulate the blood supply and make it respond more quickly. He explained that chemo changes the shape of the follicle and the colour, so it would probably grow back thicker and healthier but maybe not blonde any more. Hmmm!

ADVICE: THE 'ICE CAP'. Richard advised me that, if I had the ice cap and it fell out patchily, to shave the whole head and start again. I remembered what Paul, the Marsden wig master, had also told me about the cap but decided I would give it a whirl anyway – some hair is better than no hair!

THURSDAY 19TH JULY:
Chemo Consent

I went to the hospital to sign my chemo consent form. I was absolutely trembling but was cheered up by having lunch with my cousin Peter Lilley and his long time mate Martin Brewer at Motcomb's. The boys treated me to delicious lobster and champagne and I was feeling no pain by the time I left!

David Goodman came round later and gave both Adele – who had suffered a bad burn while cooking for us one evening, God bless her – and me some of his magic healing, which made me much calmer on the eve of my big day of first chemo. David said I should still have the chemo and surgery if I felt right with it and keep the healing as a complementary treatment but he felt that I had definitely improved since the last time he had seen me.

Luckily my husband Jeremy is very stoical and, having sadly lost his father, his brother-in-law and more recently his mother to cancer, he had seen it all before. So I did not have to stress about him. As I ate my Last Supper before chemo I remembered vividly 'Uncle' David's lung cancer and my sister-in-law Mandy standing in her kitchen patiently sieving all his fresh food through sacking. They had tried everything for David – seeing specialists all over the world. But he had died when he was younger than me, leaving Mandy with their five sons, our nephews.

Jeremy had lost his dad when he was very young but he had told me, 'I will never forget the day my father died.' Then just over a year ago his wonderful mother Sheila, 'Granny', had died. Luckily she had gone very quickly once diagnosed but I remember her at the end, dignified as ever but skinny as a rake with her distended stomach, sipping some disgusting potion while the rest of us tucked in to her delicious sandwiches. We all miss her very much; just recently Mandy had been clearing out her belongings and had sent on a letter Jade had sent from school when she was 11. It was all about school classes and eating sausages and chips and really very mundane but Jade was so pathetically pleased that her Granny had kept it all that time!

I felt very sad and maudlin that night but, thinking about how so many of our loved ones had suffered and died, I determined to gird up my loins and be strong – I was being given a life-saving treatment and it does not matter if it is a bit painful and unpleasant. Luckily Adele was there and kept my mind off things, the dear girl.

FRIDAY 20TH JULY:
First Chemo – OMG!

As Adele drove me to the Marsden Medical Day Unit (MDU) in her comfortable old Jaguar for my first chemo session I was a bundle of nerves and could hardly speak. I was truly terrified, wimp that I am. Adele chatted away happily about all sorts of things and I grunted occasionally.

ADVICE: BEFORE STARTING CHEMO. Thinking about it afterwards I recommend visiting your chemo unit before the first day.

I had envisaged being in a bed in a small dark room all by

myself with wires trailing out of me and no one to talk to. Nothing could be further from the truth at the Marsden MDU; the whole set up is very cosy and reassuring. It is open plan with each chemo chair and machine separate, so patients have some degree of privacy, but very busy and cheerful with windows all around and nurses bustling about keeping an eye on you at all times. Each chair has a laptop for your use, either to watch a film or TV or to work on and there are chairs all around for your friends and family to sit on.

The reason I had chosen to start on a day when Jade was away on holiday was because I didn't want her with me if the treatment was truly awful. But it wasn't. I think chemo is a bit like childbirth, where people will tell you all their gory details but it's not necessarily like that for you. Nowadays at the Marsden they have got it down to a fine art and you have the least possible pain and distress.

Adele came in with me as my 'chemo buddy' and she was brilliant, chatting away and taking my mind off it all. I'd had my blood test previously to make sure my blood count was strong enough to withstand the chemo. So, after having my temperature taken and being weighed, I took my promised Lorazepam and then it was time to choose a vein to cannulate. I swallowed hard and gritted my teeth as a very gentle and pretty Asian nurse (I think her name was Moto) examined my veins and chose the biggest vein in the back of my left arm, as I am mainly right handed. She put the anaesthetic cream on the vein and then covered it with a transparent plaster. Then we would wait half an hour for the gel to 'take' before 'getting the needle'. The Lorezapam was already starting to work and I found myself laughing hysterically at things – obviously high as a kite! There were some good-looking male medics around and, as my house-mate Adele is a single gal, I kept pointing them out: 'Hot doc at 9 o'clock', I'd hiss and dissolve into fits of laughter!

Mine was a morning appointment and it was quite quiet in the unit. There were a few patients dotted around, mainly women, but I could not see anyone wearing the dreaded ice cap.

Then my half hour was up and it was time for the cannula, which would 'deliver' the drugs into my system, to be inserted. I was pretty mellow from the tranquiliser so when the pretty Asian nurse returned and gently inserted the cannula into the chosen vein in my arm, I hardly felt it – just a tiny prick. No drugs yet as they would put the ice cap on first and give it time to work before administering the drugs through the cannula.

Then another very gentle, sweet-faced nurse called Beth took over. Beth was my dedicated chemo nurse and would stay with me all the way through while all the drugs were administered, I learned. She put the ice cap on – actually two caps, one on top of the other and freezing cold, naturally – with some gauze to protect my forehead and ears. At first it felt really heavy and freezing and uncomfortable on my nice warm head and I didn't think I would tolerate it but after about ten to fifteen minutes my head had cooled down and I decided to grin and bear it. They had to change it twice to keep the temperature freezing but gave me a blanket and a little heated pad to keep the rest of me warm.

About forty-five minutes after the cap had gone on (to give it time to freeze my hair follicles, so less blood flowed through them and less of the chemo reached them), Beth started to put the actual drugs into my vein. She explained exactly what she was doing every step of the way, which was reassuring.

Firstly she put an anti-nausea steroid drug in to stop me feeling sick, then Cyclophosphamide, the 'C' of 'EC', then Epirubicin, the 'E' of 'EC', and finally a saline solution to wash all the actual drugs out of my vein. She continuously checked that I had no pain or discomfort and at one point said: 'With this one, you may get a sensation as if you're sitting on a prickly hedgehog!' In fact I felt no prickles whatsoever but her phraseology made me hoot with laughter.

After all the drugs and saline had been administered I had to wait about another half an hour for the last ice cap to work, then I was finished. Rudy from the pharmacy came round to give me the three types of anti-nausea pill I was going home with and then we were free to leave.

It really hadn't been too bad. They had come round with food and drinks and newspapers and the whole experience had been as comfortable as possible, thanks to the very gentle and efficient nurses in the MDU (and the general atmosphere of calm in the unit).

Adele drove me home, fed me some of her famous homemade chicken soup and I then found that I had a window of about four or five hours when I was able to finish off my emails on the computer before I started feeling nauseous.

The three anti-nausea pills were called Dexamethasone, Ondimet and Domperidone which, like countless other cancer patients and buddies before us, we named Dom Perignon! I had to complete the course of the first two within the first three days and then take the DP as needed. The good news was that I did *not* vomit at all, which was wonderful. I started feeling nauseous at around 5pm and retired to bed surrounded by my pills and my usual supplies for nausea and dodgy tummy, namely rice cakes and Old Jamaica Ginger Beer – not exactly on the Cancer Diet! I had been told not to worry too much about the diet while on chemo and just eat like mad to keep my weight up to tolerate the treatment but I found it quite hard to eat much while feeling queasy. The rice cakes worked well and I found I was also able to eat some bananas.

One of the pills was making me feel sleepy but that was all right because I was happy to get some rest. I had a bit of insomnia later but took a Stilnoct (a mild sleeping pill from my GP) and read when I woke up at night.

SUNDAY 22ND JULY:
Recovering From Chemo – And Sue Van Colle

I stayed in bed feeling a bit nauseous but not too bad, with my meds and supplies and just read, watched TV and relaxed, with poor Jeremy looking after me as Adele had gone home. Happily he did not have to do too much as I was not up to any cooked food yet, just rice cakes, bananas and ginger beer. But he ferried these up and downstairs for me and was most solicitous.

Sue Van Colle, the Musical Director of *Carry On Brighton*, rang and told me that when she had suffered from breast cancer a few years ago, she too had had chemo first to shrink the tumour. Sue said that hers *had* shrunk and she had only needed to have a 'segmented' mastectomy instead of a total one. She said she didn't remember many side-effects – her hair had thinned but had grown back. I so hope my lumps will shrink.

MONDAY 23RD JULY:
'Crystal' And David And Ina

I had finished the course of the two pills I had to take and was onto just the Domperidone to control whatever nausea I had left, which was now quite mild. So, off to the Marsden hairdressing department where Gill fitted me with my 'Crystal' wig. I chose the 'Swedish blonde' colour, which I thought was very glam and I soon learned to brush the wig into a very natural looking style that I could wear at all times.

The good news was that, when I went to the Pharmacy to pay for the wig (only £59 on the NHS as opposed to the usual retail price of £180, I believe) I was told that as an NHS cancer patient I could fill in a prescription exemption form so that I didn't have to pay for any of my medications whilst sick. Brilliant – 'I'll have everything, please – tranqs, sleepers, painkillers, weed!'

When I dropped some books off for the outpatients' book stall, I noticed a patient having a tuna and ham sandwich, which sounded weird but I tried it and loved it. My medical team had told me to eat as much as possible and keep the calories up during chemo to help keep the side-effects at bay, and who was I to disagree? I knew that they would give me supplements if I couldn't eat but it's always much better to have proper food if you can.

While at the hospital I bumped into old friends David and Ina Bond. Ina, a glamorous mother of four, had been diagnosed with cancer about 15 years before and had miraculously kept going through various different cancers. She was quite amazing and inspiring, going on regular holidays, socialising, always looking perfectly groomed and brown as a berry. She was one of only two of my girlfriends that my husband thought good-looking (the other being Angie Best) and she still looked great but had a very swollen stomach, which she'd come to have drained, along with a blood transfusion. We arranged to have lunch soon but I realised she was going through so much more than me and that I must just get through mine without complaining too much because I'm not nearly as ill as some poor people. It's all relative.

TUESDAY 24TH JULY:
Diet And Dental Hygiene

I managed to play tennis with James, James and Jeremy today, which pleased me. I was quite tired and dizzy by the end but felt a sense of achievement for getting through it. My medical team had encouraged me to keep going with my life as much as possible whilst still getting enough rest but I was worried about nutrition because all I'd been able to manage in my first three nauseous days were rice cakes and the odd banana washed down with lashings of ginger beer – even pure water made me feel sick.

I had a phone consultation with the Marsden dietician, who encouraged me to pursue a healthy, balanced diet to keep my weight up once I'd got over my initial nausea but confirmed that I should give up most of my supplements while on chemo. I was worried about this, knowing what my immune system had been like recently, and booked up a phone consultation with the Marsden pharmacist as well.

Later I went to see my dental hygienist, Susannah at Lund Osler. Susannah had treated many chemo patients and knew I was likely to get mouth and tongue ulcers and cracked lips from chemo. My throat was also feeling sore and I felt I was already getting a nasty infection. Susannah was very gentle and recommended a Sensodyne toothpaste, softer toothbrush, thinner dental picks, an easier flossing method, gargle for my sore throat, straws for drinking and a mouthwash for the ulcers when they arrived (which they did!)

WEDNESDAY 25TH JULY:
My 5th And Worst Day After Chemo

Today was the day when I was really in pain and discomfort and thought, 'I really can't stand this for five months – what's this £20,000 treatment of Janie's in Germany when the chemo is just given to the tumour, not the whole body?'

My glands and throat were swollen up like footballs and I couldn't swallow, eat or drink. My stomach was also swollen and painful from constipation (which lasted seven days in the end), in spite of having taken everything available in my bathroom cupboard for it. And I'd had to take two sleeping pills at different times during my restless previous night.

I rang Mel at the Marsden and she suggested I go to my doctor to get antibiotics. So I dragged myself off and saw sympathetic lady doctor Dr Jourdier, in Dr McKeown's absence. She prescribed the antibiotic Amoxicillin and said it would take twenty-four to forty-eight hours to work. She also said this might just happen the first time, due to the shock to the system of chemo.

That evening was the birthday party of one of Jade's best friends, Chantelle. It had been organised by her mum Denise and our PR Charlotte at the Avista Bar at the Millennium Hotel. I knew how hard the girls had been working on the party and really didn't want to let them and Jade down, so I threw on a new frock Adele had given me and we got ourselves there, although I was feeling pretty rough and could only eat a couple of pretzels.

My friends Annie McKale, the hotel's PR, and Edward Lloyd, the OK! photographer, both said I was looking extremely fit and I suddenly realised a big truth: I wouldn't get any sympathy if I continued tarting myself up while ill!

I had a long chat with our friends Rene Azagury and his wife Rachel Elbaz and Rene told me that he had had to have chemo all through the night every three weeks when he'd had stomach cancer three years ago. He'd later had successful surgery and whipped it but still remembered those dreadful long chemo nights vividly. I could be so much worse off.

THURSDAY 26TH JULY:
R.I.P. Angharad And Mary

My glands and throat were still sore, so I rested and caught up with the papers. I was very sad to read that two popular actresses, Angharad Rees and Mary Tamm, had recently died of cancer in their early sixties. May they rest in peace. If only we spent less money on the wretched space programme and more on cancer research to keep the human beings on *this* planet alive.

In the afternoon I staggered up to my local high street with Jade to watch the Olympic flame being carried past and take some photos and mingle with the neighbours. Hopefully I will feel better tomorrow.

FRIDAY 27TH JULY:
The Olympics Open

Hooray – my glands are down and I can swallow at last! I was able to do a short radio interview and generally felt better. For the first time since my chemo I ate a proper, oven-cooked dinner at home. Then I watched the Olympics opening ceremony, which was magnificent and inspiring and took my mind off my woes.

SATURDAY 28TH JULY:
Peter Cox On Liquids

You're supposed to drink plenty of liquids, especially water, to flush out the chemo toxins, but water was giving me stomach acidity.

ADVICE: I spoke to nutritionist Peter Cox, who explained that water could bubble up and give you acidity. His advice was to drink as many other drinks as possible, especially juices, including bottled ones if necessary. I used to favour flavoured water but this is not great because of the sugar content. Jade has been making me fresh fruit smoothies in our juicer and these are excellent – and fresh veg smoothies are even better.

I spoke to Lisa, the pharmacist at the Marsden, about my previous – now dumped – supplements and she said she would send me the full report in two weeks. Like her colleague, she thought my throat infection, now cured by the antibiotics, might be a one-off due to the shock to the system of the first chemo and that my immune system would later learn to cope.

SUNDAY 29TH JULY:
Mouth Ulcers And Dreams

I've developed a new and exciting infection! As hygienist Susannah had warned, my mouth and tongue were getting sore yesterday and today I developed some nasty little ulcers. It felt as if I was eating pineapple all the time, although the Difflam mouthwash Susannah had given me, soft toothbrush and Sensodyne toothpaste are helpful. I also have bleeding cracks in my mouth and am treating these with Cetuem SCR Gold Serum.

Apparently, different patients get infections at different periods of time during the first two weeks after treatment. My throat infection happened on the fourth to fifth day and this mouth and tongue problem arrived on the ninth day. Luckily, this phase didn't last long, possibly aided by the Amoxicillin antibiotic?

I've been having Glorious Technicolor anxiety dreams on chemo, too (an accepted side-effect apparently). I have a recurrent nightmare that I can't get back from somewhere, and I also had a really vivid dream where I was being held by the Mafia at gunpoint!

MONDAY 30TH JULY:
Billy's Story

My longtime friend Billy Carter rang me. Billy was one of the first snappers I'd worked for when I first started 'moduling' in the 70s. He'd later gone on to directing as well and directed an hilarious telly show I presented called *How To Marry A Millionaire* which we shot in Florida (as one does!) Poor Billy had been diagnosed with cancer of the lymph, liver and oesophagus two years earlier and given just four months to live. However, here he was! How had he done it?

He said that after being treated at the Royal Free in Hampstead, and the Marsden, the cancer had totally vanished from his liver and there was just a bit in the lymph and a minuscule amount in the oesophagus. However, he'd had to have chemo all day, including a bag around his neck all weekend, pumping in the drugs, which was removed each Monday. He said the pills had controlled the nausea quite well but that he'd got very dehydrated, and suggested drinking at least two to three pints of liquid daily.

ADVICE: If, like me, you have the acidity and 'bubbling up' problems, just sip your liquids. Billy also advised me to eat apricot kernels daily as apparently there is some sort of

*natural arsenic in apricots that kills cancer. I immediately got
all the family munching apricots and was left with several
stones but no nutcrackers to get at the kernels! One for the
health food shops I think.*

My glands/throat were still swollen and sore, so I tottered
off to the doctor to get another five-day course of Amoxicillin. The doctor later said she should have given me a
blood test before doling out more antibiotics but luckily
forgot – hooray, I'm still not keen on the whole needle
thing, although much calmer after my hypnotherapy and
the gentleness of all my doctors and nurses.

TUESDAY 31ST JULY:
Tumour Pain

Today I noticed my tongue and mouth ulcers are healing –
due, presumably, to the antibiotics and mouthwash – and
the Cetuem Gold Serum has healed the cracks in my mouth.
Last night my tumour was hurting and I rang nurse Mel in
a panic but she said that it was either the chemo killing it or
all the proddings and tests it had received. In any case, she
reiterated, it could *not* be growing whilst I was having
chemo. She said not to worry about a blood test before the
second lot of antibiotics if I wasn't feeling too bad. Good!
Re the antibiotics, Mel said that my immune system would
start to rebuild itself immediately after finishing the treatment. It would take six months to get all the chemo out of
my body and the drugs would go on working for a month
after finishing treatment. Therefore I would not have

surgery until that month was up. It looked like I would have Christmas off, thank God – what a Christmas present it would be if the wretched thing had shrunk to nothing...

THURSDAY 2nd AUGUST:
Sharon's Story

I had my lashes done at Jinny Lash and chatted to Sarah, the receptionist. She has been very sympathetic, having had a close friend who had chemo for throat cancer. Sarah said that her friend Sharon had had a terrible time after being misdiagnosed several times. Eventually the medics got it right and she had then had chemo and successful surgery. Sarah pointed out that breast cancer patients are fortunate inasmuch as we can have mammograms to detect tumours. I guess cancer is harder to find in the throat.

FRIDAY 3RD AUGUST:
First Hair Loss?

I found more hairs than usual on my brush and think my hair's shedding, in spite of the ice cap. Jade tried to calm me down but I was in panic mode. I've got my gorgeous wiggly but was sad for my own hair and will watch it like a hawk now.

SATURDAY 4TH AUGUST:
I Stopped Feeling Sick!

Today I stopped feeling sick! It's been fifteen days since my treatment and it was just such a relief not to have to reach for the Domperidone today.

I had a dreadful nightmare last night. I dreamed that someone was punching me in the tumour and then it morphed into my usual anxiety dream of not being able to find somewhere. Obviously I'm stressed – who wouldn't be at this juncture – but, hey, I'M NOT FEELING SICK!

MONDAY 6TH AUGUST:
Paradise, Art And Simone de Beauvoir

Lucien came round to give me another hypnotherapy session. He told me to imagine a beautiful paradise for my secret go-to place and my mind came up with a mixture of St Lucia (where I'd spent my honeymoon), Jamaica (which I'd visited to heal after my dad died) and Atlantis in the Bahamas (my after-chemo dream spot). It was a really good session and afterwards I felt calmer than ever. Luce was delighted to hear how well I'd got through my first chemo.

In the evening I went to an art exhibition by some of Jade's friends and really enjoyed myself. It was bliss to be able to have a glass of wine and eat all the yummy canapés without feeling sick and I loved the 'art', buying a cute doggy drawing for my US pal Steve's birthday. As Simone De Beauvoir allegedly wrote in her Wartime Diary: 'In one sense (illness) makes every moment I live so precious; never have I felt things so profoundly'. I am definitely appreciating even little things more at the moment.

TUESDAY 7TH AUGUST:
Mother Rytasha

The inspirational Mother Rytasha, the founder of 'my' charity Food Relief International (for which I am British Chairman), rang to cheer me up. She said that laughter is absolutely the best cure, told me lots of jokes and promised to keep me supplied with more.

I'd done an interview for the Daily Express Health page and that was published today. I was pleased with it and am happy to be getting my word out there.

WEDNESDAY 8TH AUGUST:
Meds 'n' Wigs

I had a blood test and an appointment with Professor Smith at the Marsden. I related all my side-effects in gory detail and was prescribed extra pills for my stomach and insomnia. The Prof was very reassuring and measured my tumour and said it looked like it had shrunk already!

It's funny: at the hospital half the lady patients are walking around in various stages of baldness and others have perfectly coiffed big hair, obviously wigglies but gorgeous. I am almost looking forward to unleashing my Crystal on an unsuspecting world!

THURSDAY 9TH AUGUST:
Tests And 2nd Chemo

This morning Jade and I were back at the Rapid Diagnostic and Assessment Centre (RDAC) where I go to Mr Gui's clinic and for my ultrasound scans, to have a core biopsy for clinical research nurse Yukie Kano's Chemonia Research which I had signed up for. Yukie is testing how chemo affects cancer tumours. The Prof reckoned my aggressive, fast-growing type of cancer would respond well to chemo and I was interested to see the results of the core biopsy. I had agreed to take part in both Yukie's and Dr Turner's research campaigns as I believe that research today helps cancer patients of the future. You have to put something back. Kind staff nurse Elena says I am putting something back just by having cancer but that is not enough.

Yukie is very sweet and held my hand in my last blood test, even though she is an important research lady. The core biopsy was not very painful and I felt positively saintly for doing my bit for research! Then I had an ultrasound (painless) with Dr Allen and Lindsay and they told me MY TUMOUR HAD SHRUNK – quite a lot! In fact they reckoned it had gone down from nearly 3 centimetres to around 1.7 to 1.8 centimetres. This is amazing and made all my uncomfortable (let's face it, they weren't really painful!) side-effects worthwhile.

The doctor inserted a 'tumour marker' so that if the tumour shrinks a lot they will still be able to find it for inspection of the area and removal of any 'straggler' cells during surgery. Like the core biopsy, the insertion of the marker was just a bit uncomfortable, very quick and so well worth it.

I rushed off to get Jade, who was waiting in the car, and tell her my wonderful news – and bumped into my friend Nola Fontaine. She had been having treatment at the Brompton Hospital next door, so later she popped in to see Jade and we had a little catch-up in the MDU, where everyone is very relaxed about friends and family accompanying patients. Nola was looking very attractive with big hair and lippy and agreed with me that 'you don't get any sympathy if you don't look ill!' Never mind, we decided it was good to keep up our standards.

I had turned up for chemo at the usual time but was kept waiting for treatment till the afternoon. I did not know why but later discovered that my blood test yesterday had shown that my blood count was too low to tolerate chemo. So they had given me another blood test when I came in today, waited for the results and then proceeded with treatment once they saw that my blood count was now high enough for chemo. 'What a difference a day makes'! However nobody had told me what was going on – I guess because they did not want to worry me. I had had my Lorazepam so was pretty mellow, but I felt bad for Jade, who was understandably anxious about me, and sent her off to get something to eat.

ADVICE: *Ask for the results of tests each day if they impact on something else the following day. Forewarned is forearmed! And don't be frightened to ask what is going on if you are left in the dark and do not understand a situation. Some patients prefer not to know but personally I always feel better if I am in possession of all the facts, especially if another person is affected.*

I was prepared for the drugs and the ice cap this time and Jade took it all quite well. We did crossword puzzles to keep my mind off things, especially my freezing head! Jade looked around and noticed that there was only one other person having the ice cap that day: well, that was one more than last time, when I had been treated earlier and there were fewer patients. She also noticed one lady who had to have the chemo for seven hours on end. I am *so* not going to complain about my lot!

When I took the ice caps off, a huge chunk of long blonde hair came off with them. Both Jade and I gasped and I had to sit down rather quickly. Not wishing to upset the other patients, I stuffed my remaining hair into my baseball cap and left. It was 5pm and we'd been at the hospital all day, so it was time – but now I was anxious about my hair as well as what side-effects I would get this time. When I went to bed that night, I tied it up off my face in my usual 'pine-apple' (in a couple of scrunchies on top of my head so that the long ends looked like pineapple leaves – or so Jeremy says!) and left it alone. Bad mistake!

FRIDAY 10TH AUGUST:
My Friend's Stomach Cancer

I hardly dared touch my hair but was feeling sick so I just stayed in bed anyway. However, I did not feel as nauseous as the previous time, which was encouraging. My mind was taken off my troubles by a call from a long-time actress girlfriend who'd been through stomach cancer. Her situation sounded much worse than mine.

She'd been diagnosed at age 49 and the cancer was already Stage 4 (Stage 5 is basically death.) She said she'd been treated at different hospitals and had had massive surgery. At one stage she had had a haemorrhage and 'died'.

The doctors had had to tell her poor husband, but then had miraculously resuscitated her. She spent 3 and a half weeks in hospital after surgery, followed by 9 months of chemo, when she'd had to have the treatment for 3 days at a time, followed by 10 days off. The poor girl, I just couldn't imagine being hooked up to the drugs for 3 days and nights on end, she must have been so brave.

She said the treatment was like being in a tunnel with rats and spiders for ages but then one day, there was a faint light at the end of the tunnel and things started to get better. Her side-effects had included bad mouth ulcers and some hair thinning but she'd been able to cover the thinning bits with an Alice band.

Now she is completely cured, working again and happy. Interestingly she believes IVF treatment may have triggered the cancer. She said she can never drink alcohol again after her stomach cancer but it's a small price to pay for her life.

One of the hospitals where she was treated was the Marsden and she said one of the reasons they are so good there is because they have enough staff: good point.

SATURDAY 11TH AUGUST:
Things Get Hairy, And The Olympics

I felt a bit better today, so I decided to deal with my hair. For two days while I was sick in bed I'd kept it tied up in the 'pineapple' and when I took it down to brush it, it was totally unsalvageable. I'd had terrible insomnia, so I'd taken pills which had given me heavy sleeps, during which, in my anxiety, I'd obviously tossed and turned a lot. The top of the hair was OK but the back – the lengths of hair – had become a rock-solid whorl of matted hair, worse than a Rasta. It was like a huge lump of coconut matting.

Jade, Adele and I all had a go at brushing it out with detangling spray and Moroccan oil. We succeeded in brushing the top out, along with half the hair but the whorl would hardly budge except for a few straggly bits. OMG – my beloved hair, I could see I would have to have all the back of it cut off. My trusty hairdresser Steven Smith was away till Monday so I just had to be patient but we were all shocked at what had happened to it in such a short time!

Today we had Olympic tickets for the men's volleyball semi-final at Earl's Court, and I was determined to go. Jadey had gone on hols again but Jeremy, Allie and Kat accompanied me at my lethargic pace (I was less sick by the third day but had no energy at all.) All was well until the security lady asked me to remove my baseball cap. As it was now covering big bald patches and my giant whorl, I was less than keen. However, when I explained I was a chemo patient, not a terrorist, she understood completely and ushered me in.

The game, between Italy and Bulgaria, was fast and furious with Italy taking the bronze. I really enjoyed it but was dismayed to see the 'synchronised sweepers' (volunteers) who were keeping the court clean between games all had gorgeous, glossy pony tails swinging around behind their heads. Suddenly everywhere I looked there was masses of hair but not on me – I so missed my own pony tail and kept putting my hand up to feel it but it wasn't there!

We watched the Olympics closing ceremony that evening and I tried to ignore the Spice Girls' extensions and focus on

George Michael's buzz cut – very chic! I was definitely feeling much less sick this time and my stomach wasn't hurting, so I must be grateful for small mercies.

MONDAY 13TH AUGUST:
Kazzy And Victoria

I had a business lunch with my *Kazzy And Sally* TV partner Kaz, and Victoria Bullis, a dynamic American psychic and Hot Gossip contributor. Victoria is very spiritual and had been giving me healing over the phone and she said one treatment I should *not* have during chemo is acupuncture, as it 'gets everything going too much'. I had also been told I should not have massages whilst on chemo and I missed those.

Victoria suggested a visualisation technique of 'talking to the hair follicles' (very Prince Charles!) and suggested some supplements to take once the chemo was over. Visualisation is good – I'm still reciting Tatiana's mantra every morning: 'Every day in every way, I am getting better.'

The restaurant Victoria took us to was my beloved Da Mario on Queensgate Terrace and I chose a mild spaghetti vongole. I loved it but it was too much too soon on my delicate chemo'd stomach and I had really bad acidity for several days afterwards, much worse than the previous cycle. I had been told fresh shellfish was good but maybe not in a vongole! And wheat is supposed to be a stomach irritant... I was learning that I really had to respect this beast called chemo.

I'd had one particularly nice Internet comment from my

recent Daily Express piece: 'Sally's strength and spirit in hard times is very inspiring'. And Jade was always telling me, 'Be strong, Mumma'. But the relentless acidity (which went on for ten days) really got to me – it felt as if there were little rats gnawing at my guts!

TUESDAY 14TH AUGUST:
5th Day Is Worst One – Again

Today I felt so bad that I had to cancel my beloved tennis with the boys. My glands were right up and it was hurting to swallow. This time I had the Amoxicillin at hand and started the course immediately but the acidity in my stomach was horrid and one Lansoprazole (acid-reducing tablet) a day was not controlling it. Plus there was my hair...

In the afternoon my hairdresser and friend Steven Smith came over for The Night Of The Long Knives – or should that be scissors? – to cut out the dreaded giant matte. I expected to be crying like mad but it was OK because Steven was so sweet and sympathetic and took my mind off it by chatting away. He washed my poor hair and gave me a scalp massage – highly recommended – before snipping away at the offending matte, saving what he could. He cut it into a very short, boyish style, keeping the fringe (combed forward somewhat) and covering the bald patches on the top, back and sides with his expert blow drying (will I be able to do it?) I look like a schoolboy now, albeit rather a mature one. Jade later told me I looked like an elf, so I guess I'd better audition if they make any more of those Lord Of The Rings/ Hobbit fillums!

I thanked Steven so much for actually making a style out of my balding locks and he said, 'It's nothing, you've suffered enough'. (Pity the chemo doesn't think that.) All the family were very kind when they saw my shorn locks. Allie made me a lovely dinner and Jeremy actually kissed me without being instructed to – a first! Adele said I looked like Joanna Lumley as Purdey in *The New Avengers*.

News of my hair loss has spread far and wide and I had some great messages of support. A Hot Gossip client wrote, 'Go smash the chemo b....r!' and Tim, a nice chap from the Ministry Of Defence wrote, 'Here's to the return of your former luxuriant mane'. Said mane was currently sitting in the wastepaper basket because I couldn't yet bring myself to throw away the hanks of hair Steven had shorn off. So much hair, it would have filled a huge cushion. Adele thought I was mad but she also said that she was very relieved as she had thought I would have been a lot worse on chemo, i.e. vomiting, like her other friend who'd had it. It's all relative, and I must be grateful for small mercies.

When I tried on the Crystal wig over my balding bonce, I noticed there was a lot of room inside it now so much of my real hair was gone. I told Adele, 'Plenty of room for a packet of cocaine or two, I could carve out a new career as a drugs mule'. Adele replied: 'Stick to being a comedian!'

THURSDAY 16TH AUGUST:
Infections And Tears

I got the mouth ulcers and a cracked mouth again but not so bad this time and I have the curative tools to hand –

Susannah's Difflam mouthwash and Andria's Cetuem Gold Serum. Plus I'd developed another infection, which I believe would have made even my hero Charlie Sheen blush as it involved huge red lumps in delicate places. Having watched so many reruns of *Two And A Half Men* whilst ill, I wondered if it was life imitating art!

My insomnia had been awful again and I finished *A Dangerous Liaison*, the Jean Paul Sartre/Simone De Beauvoir biography my friend Katarina had given me. I shed a little tear, because that famous and brilliant couple did not believe in God so did not believe they would be reunited in Heaven. I cannot imagine not having the hope of seeing my parents and loved ones who have died once again. I know so many people are praying for me at the moment and I say my own prayers to ask for strength and light candles at our little church, St Andrew's, next door to our house. It's truly helpful to have faith to get you through hard times.

What I'm going through is so minor compared to people who are really suffering. The important thing is that I do not now think so often about dying, as I did during my time at the Charing Cross. My cancer has responded well to the chemo and I now think about beating it. I am depressed because I am insomniacal and tired and my tummy 'rats' are horrible but at least I am not vomiting.

On the news tonight Tony Nicklinson, the paralysed, 'locked in' syndrome sufferer, lost his court case to be allowed to be humanely killed. It is heartbreaking, the poor man and his family must be so desperate. He may appeal to a higher court and apparently an anonymous donor has offered to pay for him to go to Dignitas in Switzerland.

Later that insomniacal night I watched *Pretty Woman* for

the nth time and sobbed my heart out – not because the film was sad but because I knew I wouldn't have long tumbling locks like Julia Roberts again for years. Then I thought of Tony Nicklinson and shut up.

FRIDAY 17TH AUGUST:
9th Day: Feeling A Bit Better – And Anna, Martin And Mike

I took my magic Domperidone pills and trotted off to the local underground station to see if Jade, who'd done a modelling job for the Evening Standard magazine, was in it today. She was, looking ethereally beautiful as a 'dream girl' in a lacy creation. It lifted my spirits to see her and I staggered home on my bike with 20 copies, kindly dumped by travellers who only needed the paper and were blissfully unaware of my daughter's starring role in the magazine!

Today was the first day after my second bout of chemo when I was finally feeling less sick and had considerably fewer little rats running about in my entrails. I wasn't sure if this was just the cycle or because I'd switched from plain water to water mixed with fruit juice on nutritionist Peter Cox's suggestion. Amazing that pure water can make you feel worse rather than better!

I spoke to Anna Brocklebank about my acidity problem and she said that you can take more than one Lansoprazole per day safely but extra ones may not necessarily work. I determined to talk to my doctors about extra stomach medicine.

Anna told me the – ultimately uplifting – story of her

friend Martin who had had lymphoma and been treated with eight chemo sessions, one every three weeks like myself, a couple of years ago. His ex wife had insisted on moving back in to care for him and had saved his life. One night towards the end of treatment, when his immune system was at rock bottom, he'd got yet another infection and been too weak to even pick up the phone; if his wife hadn't been there to take him to hospital he would have died. Happily the couple are still together.

ADVICE: *Anna explained to me that this time while I was a cancer patient undergoing treatment was the most important time in my life because it would impact on the whole of the rest of my life. She seriously discouraged me from trying to do too much work or socialising if I wasn't feeling one hundred per cent. My medical team and many people who had been through the disease had encouraged me to get on with my life as normal as much as possible but, after listening to Anna and hearing Martin's scary story, I was chastened and decided I must maintain a balance and be very careful in the first ten days after treatment.*

Later I played back an hilarious phone message from a lady film star pal of mine who said: 'So sorry, angel – give me a ring, angel – really love you, angel – know we don't speak enough, angel.' God bless them all in Hollywood, they do cheer me up!

The next message was from my old pal Mike Winters, of Mike, Bernie and Shnorbitz fame. Mike was shocked to hear of my illness and said: 'You've always been such a healthy young lady.' Well, I was young when I first met Mike and his lovely wife Cassie in the Eighties but now I'm middle-aged and need to look after myself more carefully.

ADVICE: *I think it is very important to keep in touch with all your friends and family by phone, email, Facebook or whatever while you are ill and may not be able to actually meet people so much. Their support over the airwaves is invaluable.*

SATURDAY 18TH AUGUST:
A Wedding And A Wig

Jeremy and I had been invited to the wedding of the daughter of his friends Richard and Sally at Stowe school in Buckinghamshire and I knew he wouldn't go without me. So I popped my pills, tarted myself up and unleashed 'Crystal' on an unsuspecting Jeremy. 'Bit long, isn't it?' he said, squinting at my new golden locks and obviously having forgotten the Rapunzel extensions I'd sported for a while.

However, Crystal seemed to appeal to the younger man. When we arrived at the hotel a cute baby boy crawled after us from another room, gurgling and lifting his chubby arms towards my wiggly as I bent down to coo at him – 'Crystal' has obviously brought back my cougar appeal!

The wedding was wonderful. The Stowe School chaplain kindly alerted me as to the position of the chapel's Ladies (I had been advised to drink a lot of liquids to flush out the chemo toxins so, as when pregnant, my life now involved regular pit stops) and I was good to go. I drank champagne for the first time in two weeks, was careful what I ate and enjoyed socialising. We sat with two of Jeremy's old friends,

Mike and Jenny, who didn't bat an eye at my regular trips to the loo. I felt very tired as it was a long day but attending a glittering gathering definitely lifted my spirits.

The bride and her mum looked stunning, the speeches made me laugh and as we wandered around the beautiful grounds and admired the work of Capability Brown, I was so glad that I had used my willpower to put myself in the mood.

The next day we stopped off at the famous Bicester Village outlet stores and some retail therapy made me feel quite back to normal.

I was delighted to see Jade, who was back from her hols. She told me that my short hair looked sweet but that her friend's 19-year-old brother who had seen Crystal at the art exhibition had pronounced my wiggly hair 'cool'. Young boys, long hair... I see a pattern emerging.

MONDAY 20TH AUGUST:
Supplements And Sadness

Lisa, the Marsden pharmacist, emailed me about all the supplements I had been taking before starting chemo. She reiterated that the only ones I should take with the treatment were multi vitamins and minerals and cod liver oil and that I could also take flax seed oil pills for my eyes, which had become slightly infected this time. She said that if I ate really well I shouldn't need all the supplements. Hopefully, after I've finished chemo, the excellent Cancer Diet should see me through for life.

When I had my Jinny Lashes maintained later, Jinny said

she could see one or two gaps in my upper lashes. Uh-oh, it's starting, I thought. The second session of chemo seems to be the killer, hair wise.

The news tonight was full of the tragic death of the famous film director, Tony Scott, brother of Ridley, who had committed suicide by jumping off a Los Angeles bridge into the Pacific Ocean. A terrible tragedy. His poor family.

I had worked on a couple of commercials with Tony when I first started my career in the Seventies and found it hard to believe. People later said that he had brain cancer but his wife denied it. May he rest in peace.

TUESDAY 21ST AUGUST:
Chemo Feet And A Creepy 'Doctor'

The wedding on Saturday had tested my feet, so I visited the chiropodist, who explained that chemotherapy often affects the feet, building up hard skin. Certainly my skin seems to be very dry all over and I am slathering on the Cetuem Body Cream with reckless abandon. Strangely, two suspicious-looking but non-cancerous blemishes on my left foot seem to have improved slightly since chemo. Maybe they are drying up. Maybe I will end up looking like a prune!

I received a letter, sent to me c/o my club, The Hurlingham, from a research doctor offering to treat me. He was anti chemo, advocating nutrition and natural medicines and a treatment that he had invented which had not been taken up. I reckon, having been on the Cancer Diet and having had regular healing sessions for a while before starting chemo – which didn't shrink my tumour – that I'm doing the right thing. Personally, I think orthodox medicine combined with natural treatments and excellent nutrition is probably the answer.

(I later sent a polite email to this person explaining that I'd gone the orthodox route, combined with complementary treatments, whereupon he sent me two emails slagging off the NHS and The Ministry of Health and saying threateningly, 'It's too late [for you]. You've done it'. There really are some creeps around calling themselves doctors. A doctor has a duty of care and that does not involve scaring vulnerable patients. I sent his information on to one of my own doctors who pronounced it 'rubbish'. At least, as it turned out, the chap wasn't a member of the Club!)

WEDNESDAY 22ND AUGUST:
Brave Tony Nicklinson Dies

Today I read that Tony Nicklinson, the tragic man with 'locked-in' syndrome, who wanted to be allowed to die and had been refused by the courts, had in fact died. After the court ruling he started refusing food, fluids and medication and died six days later of pneumonia. Now he is free at last.

Later that night I was suffering from insomnia and surfing the TV channels when I came across my mate Vicki Michelle on *Celebrity Big Brother's Little Brother* and noticed that her beautiful dark hair was looking longer and glossier than ever. Consumed with jealousy I texted Vicki and received a hilarious reply. I feel blessed to have such good friends who lift my spirits. I don't have the energy to chat to them but my texting technique is much improved with so much practice!

THURSDAY 23RD AUGUST:
Hair Today, Gone Tomorrow

I did an interview with sweet Frances Hardy from the *Daily Mail* about my hair loss. That was the easy part. Next I had to be photographed with my 'comb over'! Richard Cannon, the photographer, was very nice and said I was very brave but I hated doing it, even with dear Charlotte holding my hand. I know I have to be completely honest with my readers throughout this cancer journey and show people the effects of chemo but it's difficult when you've always had a lot of hair. I am dreading the article coming out. Will I ever work again? Will people say I have good hair for radio?!

FRIDAY 24TH AUGUST:
More Tumour Shrinkage, And Tragic News About Inspirational Ina

Off to RDAC (the Rapid Diagnostic and Assessment Centre) once again for another ultrasound. Really good news: the radiologist reckons my lumps now measure only around 1.5 centimetres in total, just over half their original size. She said that, even if they totally disappeared, I will still have to have surgery with Mr Gui to remove the coil (tumour marker) and to see if there are any bad cells left. But never mind, it's going well.

After my ultrasound I went upstairs to see my girlfriend Ina, as our mutual friend, Nigel, had told me she had been hospitalised at the Marsden. Apparently her doctors had suggested moving her into a hospice but she had elected to have a special bed moved into her home in the country. Sadly she had taken a turn for the worse before that could happen.

As I walked into the private reception area of the Marsden, Ina's husband David, known as 'Bondy', was just coming in. He told me that Ina wasn't expected to last the day. I was so shocked – I simply hadn't realised how desperately ill she was. She had seemed so strong the last time I had bumped into her here.

Then David came back and said Ina wanted to see me. He said he hadn't told her what the doctors had said, so I pasted a jolly smile on my face and went in. Ina looked painfully thin and was wearing a neck brace for a new tumour in her neck (the cancer had now spread everywhere) but she still had her indomitable spirit and her lovely blue eyes were as bright as ever. We chatted about our respective hair loss, wearing evening dresses after lumpectomies and various girly things. One of her sons was there, and a girlfriend whose husband had also been treated at the Marsden, and the spacious room was full to bursting with fragrant flowers.

I didn't stay long as I realised her family would want those last precious hours alone with her. She asked me to come and see her when I returned to the hospital the following Wednesday and I of course agreed but it was a big acting job to remain cheerful. I perfectly understood why David had chosen not to tell Ina that today was the day. He and I were both crying as I left.

I hate this horrible disease that takes such beautiful people. Ina has suffered cancer so bravely for fifteen years. An amazing lady.

Later I drove down to leafy Surrey to spend a few days relaxing with my doctor friend Anna and her family. Anna is a wonderful hostess and cheers me up enormously.

SUNDAY, 26TH AUGUST:
Staying With Anna – Naima, Evva And Martin's Stories

In the paper today I read that British Army officer Naima Mohamed, who was only twenty-seven, had dropped NHS treatment in favour of 'bizarre treatments... to release bad energy' at some clinic near Harley Street. Although she had been refunded £12,000 by the clinic she had now been told that she was terminal with only two to three years to live. A terrible tragedy.

It's always good to keep an open mind but where cancer is concerned I am more than ever convinced that alternative medicine should only be used as a complement to orthodox procedures. There *are* extraordinary stories, such as that of Brandon Bays who wrote *The Journey*, but they really are the exception, not the rule.

Sadly, many people fall for the alternative stuff, especially if it's being offered on Harley Street premises, and I totally understand because chemo side-effects can be very unpleasant and surgery – being cut with knives – is not a thrilling prospect.

My healer David Goodman has always encouraged me to have the treatment the medics have offered me and use the healing to complement those treatments. My hypnotherapist Lucien Morgan says the exact same thing. That is a responsible approach.

I had also recently had an email from a friend, Evva, who said she had whipped toxoplasmosis some years ago by going on a very strict diet recommended by The Bristol Centre who had a holistic approach to cancer. She recommended a book called *The Bristol Diet* by Dr Alec Forbes. After reading *The Journey* I can understand the diet thing but you have to be incredibly disciplined. Eating like mad for chemo is very comforting and I was enjoying Anna's wonderful cooking now I was in my 'good' period.

Today Martin, the former lymphoma sufferer I mentioned earlier, came to lunch and talked to me about his experience. He confirmed that he would have died if his wife hadn't dragged him to the hospital when he caught a really bad infection near the end of his chemo treatment. Martin explained that his immune system was at zero at the end of the course – and he'd only had six sessions, not eight as I had originally thought and as I was having myself (help!). He said it would have been an easy death, just slipping away, warm and comfortable in bed. Thank God for his wife recognising how ill he was.

He'd had lymphoma all over his body – much worse than breast cancer, I realised – and bad infections throughout the chemo course. He also said he'd vomited a lot at the beginning before a kind nurse tipped him off as to the best anti-nausea drug. He was very happy and healthy now, taking great care with his diet, but had obviously been through the mill. Such a brave man.

TUESDAY 28TH AUGUST:
Warts And All

I really enjoyed the Bank Holiday weekend with Anna and co., celebrating her husband John's birthday and also their 10th wedding anniversary. Anna and I had originally planned a huge and lavish, joint wedding anniversary celebration, as my husband Jeremy and I had also been married for 10 years this year, but my darned cancer put paid to that little plan!

Anna's sons Beanie and Hamish had come down and Beanie and his girlfriend Kerry had announced their engagement and her pregnancy – all very exciting and guaranteed to take my mind off my 'helff'!

It's always good to be able to discuss your medical treatments and symptoms with a doctor who is also a friend and Anna was very patient with me. I had a little lump on one of my fingers and she warned that you can get warts whilst on chemo when your immune system is down – as during pregnancy, apparently, so we immediately warned poor Kerry! OMG, warty and balding – how attractive is that? I wonder when my hunchback will grow!

On a happier note, Anna taught me some Chi Gong (also called Qi Gong or Chi Kung) that her martial arts master had taught her. It made me feel all tingly and gave me the best night's sleep since I'd been on chemo. Can't wait to try it again.

WEDNESDAY 29TH AUGUST:
Ina: A Sad Goodbye To A Wonderful Lady

Back to the hospital for my blood test and check up before my third lot of chemo. I was hoping to visit my friend Ina again but she tragically died at 10.50 last night in her beautiful, flower-filled room, surrounded by her family. Since I had seen her on Friday she had been medically 'turned off' and lost her speech and her sight, but she had carried on for four days through sheer will power and fought bravely to the end like the true star she was. I was very sad not to be able to see her one last time but I'm relieved her suffering is over and she is at peace. My heart goes out to her husband David and their children: James, Julius, D'Arcy and Sapphire. Ina was the most inspiring of ladies, whose memory will live on.

I had my blood test with good old Freddie The Blood, the gent who has single-handedly cured my fear of blood tests (along with hypnotherapist Lucien, of course). The results were back before I saw Dr Tazia in Professor Smith's absence. She said my blood count was low again but that they would give me the chemo tomorrow, then send a district nurse round (as I would be bed bound and unable to get to my GP) to give me a 'shotty in the botty' to boost my immune system twenty-four hours later.

I was sad about Ina and worried that my immune system seemed to have gone down so quickly, and later had to have a large lunchtime drink at San Lorenzo.

Mother Rytasha, the founder of the charity I support, Food Relief International, was in London for a few days and kindly took me, Jade, her Bangladesh Number Two, Razzaque, my British co-director Claire Weldon and our British sponsor Mike Cooper to lunch. I stuck to a mild risotto, which seems to agree with my acidic stomach. We had a very happy time enlivened by a sighting of Pierce Brosnan, whom I'd named in my Hot Gossip column as 'the best looking man I have seen in the flesh'. That was some years ago but I am happy to report that nothing has changed!

Later I had a jolly dinner with the family, Adele and our nephews, James and Tom, at the local Thai restaurant. So that was two restaurant meals in one day with no bad repercussions. The end of the three-week cycle is always a good time.

THURSDAY 30TH AUGUST:
Third Chemo

I was pretty nervous about my third chemo session. The vein in my left arm had been bruised last time and was still sore, so I only had my right one to offer the nurse. Plus my blood count was low again and I dreaded another hank of hair coming off with the ice cap. However, the Lorazepam worked its magic, I had the gel on the arm, the chemo nurse Mary was very gentle putting in the cannula and Beth was again great administering the drugs.

Dr Tazia had prescribed me some Gaviscon (aniseed flavour), for my acidity as the Lanzoprazole alone simply wasn't cracking it, and Beth advised upping my soy milk intake, which should also help. I had been prescribed antibiotic eye drops as I had got an eye infection last time, which was still bothering me a bit. However, I hoped I wouldn't need to take the Amoxicillin this time as the doctor thought the booster injection would aid my immune system and stop me getting more infections.

No hair fell out with the ice cap this time and I had time to take Jade to a modelling casting and do my usual weight training at home before succumbing to the nausea and retiring to bed with my pills, rice cakes and ginger beer.

FRIDAY 31ST AUGUST:
Shotty In The Botty!

A jolly male district nurse from Nigeria, called Emmanuel, came round to give me the immune system booster injection. The 'shotty in the botty' turned out to be in the arm and wasn't too bad. Emmanuel said I was a bit dehydrated but it's tough getting loads of liquid down when you're feeling queasy in the first few days after chemo, and I'm sure ginger beer isn't a very hydrating sort of liquid! No other nasty side-effects yet though, either from the chemo or the shot.

SATURDAY 1ST SEPTEMBER:
Acidity

Once again I was feeling nauseous with a lot of stomach acidity, which felt as if I had little rats gnawing at my entrails. The Gaviscon aniseed made me feel even more nauseous, so I had to abandon that. Pure water is still giving me acidity and anything dairy makes me feel sick, so I'm sticking with the soy milk to aid the acidity problem.

Most people I've spoken to who've had chemo have had these stomach side-effects and many people think that cow's milk soothes the gut, so I asked my nutritionist Peter Cox for some advice.

ADVICE: There are no hard and fast rules on this one, says nutritionist Peter Cox. Dairy is one of many foods that irritate the gut, along with alcohol, caffeine, chillies, wheat, meat, refined sugar, fat-rich foods and raw, seedy fruits. It's certainly worth avoiding full fat milk, although natural 'live' yoghurt might be beneficial. Cow's milk is also mucus-forming, so it's probably better to avoid cow's milk and cream but instead add live yoghurt to soups and smoothies. Dill, mint and parsley in addition to ginger can assist in reducing nausea. Otherwise the rules are to eat little and often, keep to well flavoured, fluid-rich foods to reduce digestive effort and avoid naturally strong flavours which will taste 'off'. Adding salt and pepper will help stimulate your appetite and also help mask the unpleasant metallic taste associated with chemotherapy.

Happily I don't seem to have the metallic taste in my mouth and have not lost my appetite – but then my dad always said I was a 'good doer' (a term he also applied to his racehorses!)

That evening I was watching *Britain's Got Talent* when a new Bruce Willis commercial came on (I can't remember the product!) I wondered if I would get that bald and couldn't imagine the look suiting me quite as well as Mr Willis!

WEDNESDAY 5TH SEPTEMBER: *Overdoing It?*

I thought I might avoid infection this time after my immune system injection. However, true to the established pattern, my glands started swelling up yesterday, the fifth day, and it became painful to swallow. I survived by gargling for the day but didn't want to take any Paracetamol tablets for the pain, as suggested by my doctors, as they seem to aggravate my acid stomach. So today I succumbed and started another course of Amoxicillin. I was quite achey (a possible side-effect from the injection apparently) and sniffly but took my temperature on the all-singing, all-dancing, behind-the-ear thermometer I'd bought at vast expense at Boots and it was only 37.3. I knew I didn't need to be admitted to hospital, my greatest fear, unless my temperature reached 38.

Maybe I'd overdone it this time as on Monday, the fourth day after treatment, we'd had a bit of an Indian summer and I'd played tennis, gone up to Cetuem in North London for some pampering, and attended a beauty launch in the evening where I'd drunk champagne and stuffed myself with canapés (naughty naughty!). I decided I would have to limit my activities to maybe just one a day in the first week after chemo in the future.

Lots of people, including one's doctors and nurses, advise you to 'carry on with your life as normal' during chemo whereas others say 'be very careful and rest a lot'. With me there is a definite pattern of feeling grim and getting infections within the first few days after treatment, which is when I must take it easy, and then gradually getting back to normal health, and therefore activity, within the next two weeks. I certainly have very little energy in the first few days and feel weak as a kitten.

My hair hasn't shed much more after this last chemo session, just a few little bits falling out from time to time, but I have to cover my bald patches in the sun, which can really burn them. I guess Bruce Willis and other bald and balding gents get used to it but if your scalp is used to having a thick covering of hair and suddenly loses it, it will be extremely sensitive.

The Glorious Technicolor dreams are continuing. Last night I dreamt I was doing a voiceover with Demi Moore, who was looking most attractive in a turquoise Alice band and matching swirly-skirted coat dress! My dreamland is certainly more exciting than my day times at the moment. I knew that vivid dreams were a side-effect of chemo but wonder if the Temazepam is also causing them. Anyway, I think it's making me a bit dozy in the daytime so I shuffled off to my GP and got some Stilnoct, a private prescription, a lightish sleeping pill which gives you around four hours' guaranteed sleep and which I'd used safely for the odd bit of insomnia I had had in the past.

In a copied letter from the Marsden to Dr McKeown I had noted that Dr Tazia Irfan had described me as 'a pleasant lady'. Interesting. Considering my insomnia for most of the time and general discomfort for some of the time, I *am* pretty good-tempered – a combination of the hypno and the Temazepam, maybe? I decided to use the Temazepam for the first week after treatment and the Stilnoct, only if strictly necessary, for the second two weeks.

THURSDAY 6TH SEPTEMBER:
Does A Vegan Diet Help?

Today I spoke to a lady who had started chemo for cancer of the breast and lymph two weeks before me. She was very positive, said she had lots of energy (although this later slowed down) and had not really had any side-effects at all, apart from losing some hair. Amazing – this is the first person I've spoken to who is doing so well on chemo. She put it down to having gone on a vegan diet with her sympathetic husband, cutting out alcohol, sugar, red meat, etc., and going completely alkaline. Remembering Brandon Bays and my friend Evva, I absolutely get this. She said that her tumour had also shrunk by around fifty to seventy per cent and that she had also had a tumour marker inserted, like me.

Although she had never really felt ill, she had got an infection – an inflammation caused by the marker, possibly when it pushed on a cyst she had in her breast, which was later drained. The bad news was that she had had to be hospitalised and hated the experience. Although she was a private patient at the calm and comfortable Marsden, she found it extremely distressing, with all the constant tests, not sleeping and becoming exhausted, not getting her usual vegan food and not being in control of her life. She had had to stay in hospital for a week but was now happily back at home.

Coincidentally, this lady had had the same problem as me injection-wise. Her chemo entry vein had been bruised and remained so, just like mine (and it continued to be bruised and sore for two months). I can see where the PICC line could be useful if one was having chemo – and therefore blood tests – very regularly, such as every week or ten days.

She also said that she had had the 'nutropenic immune system' booster injection after each cycle. I presumed from looking at my blood test notes and spotting the word 'nutropenic' that this is what I had had. She had had the injections in her tummy and said they were completely painless in that area when the nurse gave them to her but when she had tried to inject herself, it *had* hurt, possibly due to stress.

She said she missed eating out, as there weren't many good vegan restaurants around, apart from Chutney Mary's in the King's Road, but that she now intended to 'keep the cancer gene turned off' by what she ate.

Yesterday, Sian Busby, novelist and wife of BBC Business Editor Robert Peston, died, aged 51, after a five-year battle with lung cancer. She was bravely working on her last novel right up until her death. May she rest in peace.

One of Lucien's hypno colleagues who I'd known for yonks, Susie Sylvie, kindly sent me a little book of healing and protection called *The Holy Zohar*, published by The Kabbalah Centre. I've heard of Kabbalah mainly due to Madonna and thought 'Well, it can't hurt'.

Somebody else sent me one of those chain letter prayers where, if you don't send it on, something bad will happen. That *can* harm by causing stress and is totally unacceptable. I am convinced that God does not believe in superstitious blackmail.

FRIDAY 7TH SEPTEMBER:
Support For My Hair Loss

My *Daily Mail* hair loss article was published today and I quaked in my boots as to people's reactions. However, friends and the public alike have been truly supportive and

I am now cool about wearing my hair short when it eventually grows back. Personally I don't think I am good looking enough to take short hair but will probably be fed up with the wiggly by then!

SATURDAY 8TH SEPTEMBER:
Aunty Pam And Risotto

Jeremy's adorable 93-year-old Aunty Pam had been ill with a hacking cough for some time and was admitted to hospital today. I was so sad that I wasn't able to go and see her, as chemo patients have to keep away from infectious people and situations. Oh well, only just over three months to go now.

One of Jeremy's family friends, Pat Gait, rang up to tell me how much she liked the newspaper photo of me with the 'pixie' hair. Pat is a beauty who rocks short hair and we discussed its merits – double-quick drying time for one!

Jade was stood up by one of her soppy girlfriends last night, so I'd offered to take her out tonight however bad I was feeling – mind over matter! In fact today, the tenth day, I was feeling much better and we went to Sette, Frankie Dettori and Marco Pierre White's latest swanky eaterie on Chelsea's Sydney Street, on the recommendation of our friend Matthew Steeples, who said they could make something special for me if necessary. Jade and I had been devastated when Frankie's in Chiswick had closed down recently as it was situated conveniently next door to her theatrical agency, Hobson's, and we always went there after visiting Gaynor, her agent. But the new one was great, serving a very good risotto which was easy to digest and all the staff made a great fuss of me, knowing my situation.

SUNDAY 9TH SEPTEMBER:
A New Ice Cap?

As I washed my hair (an exercise that now requires very little shampoo and conditioner) today, I noticed very little falling out and wondered what the big difference was between the second chemo (biggest fallout since Nagasaki!) and the third (hardly anything).

As I write, they have apparently started using another type of ice cap at the Marsden, one that you put on two hours before chemo so the scalp should be really and truly frozen (Michael Jackson would have approved!). I wondered if the new type of cap then stays on during the hour or so of your chemo treatment as well – and for some time after-wards, like the current one. I don't think I could tolerate three to four hours of iciness on my noddle, and that is what I am dreading when I start Taxol, which apparently takes twice as long as EC. Could be time to give up the cap and go for a big fall-out.

Looking at my face without much hair, I realised that I do indeed resemble an elf, with my slightly sticking-out ears. Should I embrace the look and dye myself green if all my hair falls out?

MONDAY 10TH SEPTEMBER:
Am I Getting A Stomach Ulcer? What Should I Eat?

As I had not been able to get hold of either the nurses at the hospital or my GP, I had booked a phone consultation with the knowledgeable Patricia Peat from Cancer Options.

ADVICE: NHS staff are always very busy, so it is good to have back-up, including private advice if you can afford it. Anyone can ring Cancer Options on 0845 009 2041, or log on at www.canceroptions.co.uk

I was worried that, with such bad acidity and some rectal bleeding, I might get a stomach ulcer and Patricia confirmed that that was, sadly, a possibility with the chemo. She said that the Yakult, live yoghurt and soy milk I was already taking were good for the gut and to also try aloe vera liquid and sodium bicarbonate. As the Gaviscon aniseed liquid had made me more nauseous, she suggested finding a similar antacid that suited me better – apparently liquid antacids are better than the chewable tablets for lining the stomach.

I also discussed the liquids situation with Patricia. I had been drinking like mad – mainly fruit and vegetable juice mixed with water – because I had felt dehydrated and wanted to flush out the chemo toxins. But all this liquid was affecting my insomnia by waking me up several times a night for calls of nature! Patricia confirmed that it is safe to drink less liquid, so I will cut it down from two litres a day to up to one-and-a-half, and nature calls can take a hike!

Patricia later sent me her definitive list of alkaline, acid and neutral-to-alkaline foods, which can be found at the back of this book. Cancer apparently cannot live in an alkaline environment and eating alkaline foods will also help with stomach acidity.

Different cancer books give different information about foods and it is very confusing. Patricia's advice tallied with that of my nutritionist, Peter Cox, and my 'roomie' Adele, who is super knowledgeable about cancer fighting foods, so this is what I trust. Adele's healthy eating daughter, Tash, advised me to try natural organic agave syrup (not heated) for sweetening. It is even more yummy than raw honey, which is also safe.

My driver, Robert Meah, who is the same age as me and extremely healthy as well as very knowledgeable about cancer, says raw courgettes, walnuts and freshly-squeezed wheat grass are also excellent at combating cancer.

My feeling – as a cancer sufferer rather than a cancer expert – is that while you are on chemo, everything bad is being killed anyway and you should eat what suits your stomach. For instance, potatoes, rice and rice cakes all soothe my stomach in my acidic first ten days of the cycle but are not officially alkaline. Once the chemo treatment is finished and my stomach gets back to normal, I will concentrate on sticking to the Cancer Diet one hundred per cent. After all, once you have had cancer you need to eat safely for life. I very much admire people like Brandon Bays who only eat raw fruit and vegetables and thus kill their tumours but it does not suit my particular stomach.

TUESDAY 11TH SEPTEMBER:
Ann-Marie's Wig Advice

I drove down to Surrey to stay with my medical mate Anna, who always lifts my spirits with her cheerful conversation and delicious cooking, and spent hours discussing all my side-effects with her patient husband John, housekeeper Michelle and T'ai Chi teacher Shelave.

While there, a long-time cancer survivor friend, Ann-

Marie, rang me. She had had a very aggressive cancer ten years ago when she was in her thirties. An extraordinarily brave lady, she had lost her beloved son Duncan two years ago to a fatal asthma attack. He was just fourteen. It was so kind of her to bother with me when she was still broken hearted.

ADVICE: *Attaching wigs. Ann-Marie had gone through chemo, lost all her hair and elected to wear a wig full time so as not to scare Duncan, who was very young at the time. She still wanted to 'look like mummy' for her little boy. She said she thought my hair would all fall out eventually and advised attaching the wig to my head at the crown, back and sides with double-sided tape once the time came. I presumed this would only work when you are completely bald or are pre-pared to wear a wig all the time, as the tape would otherwise pull even more hair out when the wig was removed. Ann-Marie also said to make sure the wig fitted really snugly before attaching it to the scalp and most wigs have elastic bits at the back which you can adjust.*

I was not so worried about losing the rest of my hair now that the best bits had already gone. Nothing could be worse than losing my long thick 'tail' – that's what I really missed and that experience had been truly traumatic. I decided not to shave the lot off as some patients do. I cannot make any sort of proper short-haired style out of my current patchy bonce, even with a 'Hamlet commercial' comb-over but my – now short and thin – bits of hair are useful for attaching the wig with grips, which is quicker and more comfortable than double sided tape.

THURSDAY 13TH SEPTEMBER:
A Message From Marilyn?

I drove back from Anna's feeling better after a relaxing stay and some fresh country air but back on the Amoxicillin with yet another throat and chest infection. Ho hum. But I was well enough to drive Jade to her London Fashion Week castings (she booked shows with four different designers, so it was worth it).

As we were driving, Jade asked me if our best friends Marilyn and Kat Lambert had been the first people to visit us at St Mary's Hospital when she was first born. As I mentioned before, Marilyn had sadly died eighteen years ago after having breast cancer herself and Kat later came to live with us.

I thought back to that time twenty years ago when I was recovering from the birth of my little treasure in the Lindo Wing at St Mary's, where all the kind nurses seemed to be called 'Mary' too.

'Yes', I replied.

Then Jade said: 'Did you just touch my shoulder?'

'No, I'm driving,' I answered.

'Well, someone did. It must have been a ghost,' she said.

'Marilyn!' we both exclaimed, at the same time.

Sadly I am not a particularly spiritual person but I like to think that Marilyn, our long-time next door neighbour and a dear friend is watching over us now.

FRIDAY 14TH SEPTEMBER:
Missing Ina's Funeral – And Old Friends

For the first time since starting chemo and getting regular infections, the Amoxicillin does not seem to be controlling my chest infection and I am sniffing and coughing and ploughing through the Kleenex. I don't think the booster boosted me enough! Even so, I tried to play tennis with my regular partner Jackie, known as Venus (I am Serena of course!) but did not have enough energy. I was fed up and made an appointment to see my GP on Monday.

I was also very sad because I had to miss my friend Ina's funeral in Cirencester. I would really have liked to be there to pay my respects to such an amazing lady but my cold was streaming today and I just wasn't strong enough to drive all the way down there and back. But I was with Ina in spirit and know she understands up there.

I got home to find a lovely message from my old mate and favourite 'stage husband' Jess Conrad, which cheered me up. It's because of Jess and an old joke we had on tour that I call hairpieces 'ferrets' (I wore one in the play at the time; he has a perfect head of hair). I would love to wear a ferret at the moment but have not got enough hair to attach one to!

Then Jade made me my daily fruit smoothie and reminded me to knock it back immediately.

ADVICE: Drink fruit and veg smoothies, wheat grass juice, etc, immediately, otherwise you lose the goodness. I tend to sip my drinks since being on chemo, as sips are easier to digest on days when stomach acid is really playing up.

113

That evening I loaded my handbag with Kleenex and joined Adele and Mike Cooper at one of my locals, The Troubadour, and ate fish soup with no dairy and sweet potatoes, both very good for me. My friend, the author Robin Anderson, who dedicated his last book to me, was there and pleased to see me *not* drinking loads of vino.

SATURDAY 15TH SEPTEMBER:
Friends With Prostate Cancer

I bumped into my neighbour, Alastair, and we compared notes about our respective cancers. He had recently been diagnosed with prostate cancer and was due to start treatment in a month. He said that one side-effect was loss of a certain function and that, as a married man, he had been given several boxes of Viagra which he was just off to trial! A very positive chap...

Then I received a nice card from a mature theatre producer friend who had liked the most recent Mail article and felt that he could now confide in me.

He revealed that he had been diagnosed with prostate cancer eight years earlier and been advised of five different possible ways to go:
1) surgery
2) chemo
3) radio
4) hormone treatment
5) doing nothing and 'living and dying with it'.

The tumour had been too big for surgery so he had opted for hormone treatment. He said he was now pronounced 'well' but that he had to live with the side-effects 'which I won't go into now'. I can certainly understand an older person not wanting to go through the rigours of chemo.

Prostate is the most common male cancer, just as breast is the most common female one, and I have sadly lost three friends to it, although I think they are getting to grips with prostate these days. I remember interviewing Bob Champion and his scientists at The Bob Champion Cancer Trust for B Well TV a few years ago and being very impressed with the research.

SUNDAY 16TH SEPTEMBER:
Aunty Pam And Hillie – And Breasts Are Everywhere!

Jeremy went off to see Aunty Pam in Surrey. He had been unable to get through to the hospital, which was worrying. We will have to get a mobile for Pam but Jeremy later said she was recovering well and should be out tomorrow, thank goodness.

ADVICE: *If your hospital is very busy and there is no one – at least no one who speaks English – on reception, ask if you can take your mobile in with you – but don't forget the charger!*

Speaking of aunts, I later received a lovely message from Hillie Marshall, agony aunt extraordinaire and one of our Hot Gossip contributors. Hillie said that she had been to Lourdes, lit a candle for me and collected water for me from the Holy Spring, which she would give me when she saw me next. That is so thoughtful; I am truly blessed with my friends and family.

Breasts are being mentioned everywhere at the moment, as is breast cancer. There has been a huge furore in the media this week after the Duchess of Cambridge was papped sunbathing topless on holiday with Prince William at Viscount Linley's chateau in the South of France. Much has been written and said about the scurrilous French paparazzi, harking back to the tragedy of the late Diana, Princess of Wales, and the Palace has taken the unprecedented step of suing *Closer*, the French magazine that first published the offending images. There has been much sympathy for poor Kate but her boobs are of course in excellent shape, like the rest of her.

Suzanne Moore wrote in her Mail On Sunday column today: 'Kate is said to be in "agony" while she and William are being unspeakably "brave"... I know women in 'agony' and who are 'brave' because they have breast cancer.'

Thank you, Suzanne.

WEDNESDAY 19TH SEPTEMBER:
Crystal, Mucositis And Alexander Monson's Memorial Service

I was all gussied up, with Crystal covering my balding head, when I went to the Marsden today, as I had a busy, smart day ahead. Elena did not recognise me without my usual hospital uniform of baseball cap and trackie bums! The blood test nurse and the doctor were very complimentary and I feel this is all down to my 'fetching' (as the *Daily Mail* described it) wig. Oh, the wonders of modern wiggery! If you look good, you feel good, no question. Dr Anandappa, the lady doc on the Prof's team who saw me this time, said she was so proud of all her patients because we all made such an effort to look chic in spite of all our hair loss and other side-effects.

I discussed my side-effect problems with her, starting off with the large vein at the back of my left arm, which had swelled up nastily after two chemo sessions and was still sore and red after six weeks. The doctor said that it would probably remain that way for a few months and I worried about the large vein in my other arm being able to last the course.

Then I mentioned my sore throats needing regular antibiotics, which both my GP and I were worried about, and my extreme and painful stomach acidity, which made me concerned about the possibility of getting a stomach ulcer. Dr Anandappa said she thought my throat problem might not actually be an infection requiring antibiotics but something called mucositis, which might be linked to my stomach acidity. This was wonderful news if true. She prescribed me a new medicine called Sucralfate (usually used to treat ulcers) and I trotted off with renewed hope.

Then it was off to the memorial service for Alexander Monson, who had been tragically killed with a fatal blow to the back of the head while in police custody in Kenya. A ghastly thing – he was only twenty-eight. Alexander's grieving father Nicholas (Lord) Monson organised a splendid service for 400 people and has started a foundation to assist victims of police brutality all over the world. All our hearts went out to Nicholas; he has been so brave.

I bumped into a friend at the reception in the church garden who had melanoma (skin cancer) on his head. He said it was quite sore and, as there was a touch of weak English sun around I chided him for not wearing a hat, remembering how sore my little balding noddle was when first inadvertently exposed to the sun. He said that luckily he did not have to have chemo or radiotherapy and was able to take pills for the condition.

Everyone said I was looking amazingly well and I thanked God for 'Crystal' and make-up allowing me to pay my respects to Alexander's memory looking respectable.

THURSDAY 20TH SEPTEMBER:
Nausea, Veins, A Goodbye, A Good Wish And A Party

For the first time, I felt nauseous during my fourth chemo session today but I think it was due to anxiety about my vein situation. Luckily the girls with the food and beverage trolley came round and I was able to buy a ginger beer, which always helps.

The efficient nurse who put my cannula in today told me that my right large vein in the back of my arm was too hard for insertion today and she would have to use the – much smaller – vein in the front of my arm. This was more unpleasant, as the lovely gentle Beth, my regular chemo nurse, had to 'push' the solutions in from time to time and I could actually feel them going in – anathema for me after my previous anaesthesia injection trauma some years ago. Thank goodness I had had the hypno sessions with Lucien Morgan to work on my trauma. That and my usual

Lorazepam saved me from embarrassing myself and my faithful Jade, who was once again holding my hand through the treatment. The ice cap was still a pretty horrid experience but I got through it and there were only a couple of hairs stuck to the cap when it was removed this time. Beth also noticed some little chick hairs growing back on my bald patches so maybe the cap is worth it.

I talked about my vein problem with Beth and wondered whether I should have the PICC line in the future. We also discussed my acidity and insomnia. Beth felt I would be better off with pear and peach juice, rather than my apple and mango mix, but that the prune and V8 juices were fine. Regarding getting up in the night to go to the loo, Beth felt I probably was drinking too much liquid, what with the green tea, soy milk and Jade's smoothies as well as the fruit juice mixed with water.

This was my last EC (Epirubicin and Cyclophosphamide) chemo session and I was pleased to be finished with it and to be halfway through my treatment. But I am scared of the Taxol (Paclitaxel), which I will be having at two-weekly intervals instead of every three weeks, as with the EC. Beth told me that the Taxol treatment takes at least two hours; that will be at least three and a half hours with the ice cap and I do not know whether I will be able to tolerate the cap for that long.

ADVICE: *If you do not have the ice cap, apparently Taxol can make you drowsy and you might be able to have a nice sleep during the treatment.*

This was also Beth's last time with me as she has been

119

made an offer she could not refuse at another hospital and is leaving the Marsden. Jade and I wished her well but I will miss her terribly.

Today was my mother's birthday and Jade and I wished her a happy birthday in Heaven. She is always with us because we carry her in our hearts and I believe that both my mother and father are looking down on me and protecting me at this difficult time. We are not a super-religious family but I like to believe in the afterlife because it gives you hope of seeing loved ones who have passed.

It had been quite a gruelling session today but I cheered myself up no end by attending my Marbella pal Marc Burca's cocktail party with Jeremy where I guzzled Pimms – definitely not featured on the Cancer Diet but I really needed it. I chatted to friends and had my photo snapped wearing Crystal by dear Edward Lloyd. Everyone was very kind to me but some people are a bit timid as to how to talk to patients about cancer and chemo. I feel it is my mission to give them as much information as possible in case they or their loved ones go through it.

ADVICE: The intelligent Ingrid Seward, editor of Majesty magazine and regular Mail contributor, advised me to 'tell people to ask the right questions'. She is so right.

FRIDAY 21ST SEPTEMBER:
Sucralfate And Sleep

The new medicine, Sucralfate, seems to be agreeing with me and coating my stomach successfully, so I did not have much acidity today. At 6pm, twenty-four hours after my chemo finished, a district nurse came round to give me my booster shot. I am hoping for an easier ride this time. I did not have much nausea today but felt extremely tired, although this could have been from the Temazepam I had been prescribed for my insomnia.

ADVICE: Beth had explained that all sleeping pills only give you around four hours of drugged sleep, so it is best to take your pill when you go to bed and let your natural sleep pattern take over for the rest of the night, rather than go to sleep naturally and take your pill at three in the morning – the time you tend to wake up if you have insomnia – as that will make you more dopey the next day.

SATURDAY 22ND SEPTEMBER:
Heather, Liz, And Advice From A Doctor And A Professor

Today I was feeling quite nauseous again. Side-effects are very up and down and you cannot really plan to do much for the first few days after treatment. By the evening, stuffed full of meds, I was feeling better but lonely by myself in the house after Jeremy had gone fishing, Allie had gone to visit his mum in Somerset and Jade was doing two nights' shooting on the new Vin Diesel 'Fast And Furious' film, playing a party girl all decked out in a 'Barbarella' type cozzi.

I decided to attend Heather Bird's dinner after her Anti-Ageing Conference at the Copthorne Tara Hotel nearby in Kensington. (I would have liked to attend the conference as

I feel that suffering cancer, and certainly chemo, must be ageing for the soul as well as the body but had not felt well enough in the daytime.) It was a lovely evening and cheered me up enormously.

Heather Bird, who runs HB Health, is an inspirational health and anti-ageing expert and always interesting to listen to. I sat next to the very wise Harley Street consultant physician, Dr John Keet, who advised me to have a PET/CT scan (which uses two forms of imaging at the same time and shows how organs are working) for my whole body privately once I had finished my treatments – just in case.

On the other side I had the very dynamic and healthy Liz Brewer, who said she had had a lot of cancer in her family and advised me to visit the Optimum Health Institute in Texas regularly once I was cured – to keep me that way.

ADVICE: *How to eat anti-cancer food, broccoli. I also chatted to one of the doctors at the conference, Professor Ron Hagadus, about the benefits of broccoli for cancer patients (much has been written in the papers about this recently) and he said that you have to chew broccoli for a long time to get all the goodness out of it: very interesting. Everyone is being very kind and helpful and I am very grateful.*

Funnily enough Liz said she had never seen me looking better and I put this down to my new hairiness! Since starting to lose both my head hair and lashes, I have taken to wearing 'Crystal' regularly in the evenings and getting myself Jinny lashed every month. Luscious locks and lashes cover up a multitude of sins and distract the eye from any paleness and under-eye shadows caused by illness, chemo and insomnia.

SUNDAY 23RD SEPTEMBER:
Fiona's Story

Today I finally got to speak to one of my tennis chums, Fiona, who had breast cancer two years ago. In February 2009 she found a lump under her arm, so her GP sent her for ultrasound at a nearby hospital. Later at her GP's surgery he told her it was an enlarged lymph node containing fluid. He asked what she wanted to do about it and at the time Fiona decided that she would keep an eye on it (in the hope it would go away) but if it got any bigger she would return.

One year on, in February 2010, Fiona thought the lump had got bigger so returned to her GP's surgery. Her doctor – a woman this time – referred her back to the hospital for another ultrasound and the radiographer said that it had not got bigger but it had changed shape and he advised her to get it removed. Fiona and her GP immediately agreed and Fiona had day surgery to have the lymph node excised. A mammogram produced clear results, so Fiona was not unduly worried until her surgeon called her after the biopsy to say that the lump was not an enlarged lymph node as originally thought but was in fact the tail end of the breast tissue containing 1 centimetre of invasive lobular cancer.

The surgeon said it was invasive but slow growing. This diagnosis was then followed quickly by MRI, CT and bone scans, which fortunately proved the cancer had not spread and the lymph nodes were clear. Fiona then had two further operations to try to remove the surrounding LCIS (lobular cancer in situ). However as it was impossible to obtain a sufficient clear margin, the surgeon, in consultation with

123

colleagues, decided the best result would be for Fiona to have a subcutaneous mastectomy (i.e. the skin and the nipple remain intact and they remove the inside breast tissue). Fiona's surgeon suggested reconstruction at the same time and Fiona opted not for the long, eight-hour operation using her own flesh to reconstruct (in fact not really an option at the time as the surgeons didn't think she would have enough flesh!) but for an implant and expander (as had been offered to me at the Charing Cross.)

So in June 2010 Fiona had a 'temporary', smaller implant fitted with expander and the plan was the permanent implant would be fitted a few months later. But that changed at a meeting with her oncologist in July 2010. On being found to be HER2 positive Fiona was told that she needed the drug Herceptin. Having originally thought she would get away with just radiotherapy, the need for Herceptin meant it was administered along with chemo – something that is not the case in all countries but 'best practice' in the UK. So Herceptin was given at three-weekly cycles (starting at the same time as chemo) for a period of one year. Fortunately this drug has no side-effects.

Fiona started her six sessions of chemo (along with Herceptin) at the beginning of August 2010 followed by five weeks of radiotherapy until February 2011. The Herceptin finished in July 2011 after which Fiona was put on Tamoxifen and six months later changed to Arimidex.

Chemo resulted in a few side-effects, including hair loss, extreme fatigue after sessions five and six plus some overall swelling (caused by steroids and water retention) towards the end and, in particular, numbness in the toes and fingers. Her – normally short – hair grew back to its original length quite quickly, albeit a little more grey (normal for us mid-dle-aged ladies apparently.)

Two years on from the biopsy Fiona finally had the 'temporary' implant replaced with a permanent one in February 2012 – radiotherapy needs time to settle so it was thought best to wait a year before doing the final op.

She sounded very cheerful, quite back to normal, and advised me that, despite initially being in a dark place and not maybe seeing it at the time while going through the treatments, there is definitely 'light at the end of the tunnel'.

All that's left is Arimidex for five years, six-monthly check ups with her surgeon and oncologist, and annual MRI scans. It had taken two years of her life in total. A brave lady.

MONDAY 24TH SEPTEMBER:
Family Time And A Friend's Bad News

My brother and sister-in-law had arrived back from their beautiful home in Italy looking brown as berries and we had a jolly family dinner at The Troubadour.

'Aunty Caroline' had filled me with hope when she had told me about a lady they had heard of, an employee's aunty who was apparently 'sailing through' chemo, continuing to work the whole time. However, she told us tonight that the poor lady had recently collapsed on a station platform and been carted off to hospital. It's official – I have not found a single chemo patient who has not either had bad side-effects or eventually been hospitalised while on the treatment. You have to have tremendous respect for, and a healthy fear of, these chemicals that are being pumped into you and not push yourself too hard.

ADVICE: Losing work whilst on treatment. Patients can apply for benefits if they are too ill to work and do not have adequate savings.

TUESDAY 25TH SEPTEMBER:
Bloody Tuesday

This morning as I walked into the bathroom in my nightie I saw a large drop of bright red blood on the floor – then another – and another – and another... OMG, I was bleeding from my backside! The blood was dripping down and staining the cream carpet – my husband would be most upset!

In spite of Lucien's helpful hypno sessions, I still cannot stand the sight of blood and I practically fainted, gripping the side of the bath. Hyperventilating and trembling like a leaf, I rang the nurses' line at the hospital and booked a phone consultation with my GP on duty.

I have to say, if there is something serious the Marsden machine goes into action fast. Within five minutes, Helen, one of the sympathetic nurses, rang back and within fifteen minutes I was speaking to Dr Anandappa, whom I had seen last time.

ADVICE: For future bad chemo side-effects I was told to ring the medical day unit (MDU, chemo unit) at the hospital, as they are in charge of all chemo treatments and chemo related

problems. This was what I did the next time I had a crisis —
which sadly was not too far away!

Dr Anandappa confirmed what I had read: that this (having blood drip out of your butt for no apparent reason) was a normal chemo side-effect – blooming terrifying though! She was very sweet and said that, if I had not lost more than a tablespoonful of blood, it was not dangerous and was probably just haemorrhoids, which are normal with chemo. She suggested I apply some haemorrhoid cream (I actually had some of this, as it is supposed to get rid of wrinkles!). Although I had never noticed any improvement of the wrinkles on my elbows (the only place I had dared to try it), the haemorrhoid cream may now come into its own!

Then my lady GP, Dr Cole, rang me and she also reassured me and said I could come in the following day if I had not stopped bleeding. (Happily the bleeding stopped quickly and did not bother me again for the rest of the chemo course.) I got down to scrubbing the carpet with a nail brush but felt queasy all day – I just hate the sight of blood. I am such a wimp!

Dr Anandappa had also advised me that I could stop taking the Sucralfate as soon as my acidity ended. That was great news as although it was working well with lining the stomach I felt it was making me even more dehydrated than usual.

WEDNESDAY 26TH SEPTEMBER:
Louisa, And Preparing For 'Breast Cancer Awareness Month'

I cancelled tennis today as I was feeling exhausted and nauseous. My tennis partner James' wife Louisa said she could not understand how I could play at all. She said she had 'just collapsed' while on chemo some years ago. I do think chemo is much easier to tolerate these days – I believe the medics have learned with experience how to keep chemo patients more comfortable. Happily Louisa is now fine and a demon on the tennis court once again!

Later in the day I managed to drag myself, with Charlotte, to Kazzy's studio to do a shoot for Cancer Relief UK for the upcoming Breast Cancer Awareness Month (October). Asda and Interflora were donating the full cost of floral bouquets bought during the month to the charity and I posed with a colourful bouquet for the cause. I felt sick as a dog and sipped ginger beer all the way through but Charlotte and Kaz were very understanding and the pics looked great.

I had bad acidity during the – usual insomniacal – night but both that and the nausea seemed better the following morning. I feel the Sucralfate is helping.

THURSDAY 27TH SEPTEMBER:
Off To 'Marbs'!

The doctors gave me permission to go on holiday – hooray! So it was off to Marbella to visit my close friend and Jade's Godmum, Patricia 'Aunty Pat' Duncan, and her doggy Pasha, whom she had kindly shared with Jade during her school-days. Our clever travel agent Nigel Dean, after many years of travelling with cancer patient extraordinaire Ina Bond, suggested 'wheelchair assistance' as there is a fifteen-minute walk to the gates at Gatwick. This sounded a bit serious but turned out to be a neat buggy driven by a lovely British Airways lady called Sabina, and Jade and I loved being whizzed around the airport in style. There are definitely some advantages to being ill!

However the plane was diverted to Seville due to bad weather in Malaga, the air conditioning was fierce, there were no blankets and a large gentleman in the row behind us was snorting and hawking disgustingly. So, in spite of donning all the clothes we had with us, Jade and I were sniffling by the time we finally got rerouted to Malaga.

ADVICE: *Although some sun and Vitamin D is good for you, do not attempt a holiday in a sunny climate unless the sun is guaranteed. You cannot afford to catch a cold that might develop into a more serious infection requiring hospitalisation. Take warm clothes to travel in even if visiting a hot country.*

I had been advised to travel Business/Club Class as there are fewer potentially germ-ridden travellers around you but the germs are mainly carried in the air conditioning so you take your chances in any Class.

My acidity and nausea were better today in spite of being separated from my Sucralfate bottle for several hours whilst flying around Spain because it contained more than 100 ml and couldn't go in my hand luggage. I believe having something nice to concentrate on, like a trip, takes your mind off your side-effects – mind over matter.

FRIDAY 28TH SEPTEMBER:
Justin's Story – A Mother's Faith

Funnily enough, poor Jade is suffering much more than me with sore throat and swollen glands, whereas I seem to have escaped it this time – due to the Sucralfate, the booster or both? I feel dreadful for her and wish it was me, as I am now used to it. Luckily she is getting over it quickly. The weather was rainy but we cheered ourselves up with some 'retail therapy' in the famous Marbella shops!

In the evening Pat's friend Dalene came over and told me the inspirational story of her son Justin. When he was just seventeen, poor Justin was struck down with meningococcal meningitis and Dalene was told he only had five days to live. But she stayed with him day and night in the hospital, praying to Our Lady and Saint Jude and clutching her Saint Jude medallion. A miracle occurred and Justin woke up and made a complete recovery although the doctors had said that, even if he lived, he would be blind and paralysed. Dalene put his extraordinary recovery down to her belief and the power of prayer. Justin is now thirty-five, fit and healthy!

She asked me to touch the famous Saint Jude medallion and said she would add me to her prayer list. Pat is also praying for me every day. I am so blessed in my friends.

SATURDAY 29TH SEPTEMBER:
Valerie's Story

Pat's friend Valerie rang. She had had breast cancer two years ago and, after successful surgery and radio, was now on Tamoxifen for five years. Valerie said she had thankfully avoided mastectomies but had had lumpectomies in both breasts, plus lymph removed from both sides, followed by radiotherapy for five weeks, but luckily no chemo. She said the surgery scars were very small and the breasts had no visible 'dents', so she was very happy with the results.

However, she had gained twenty pounds in weight since being on Tamoxifen, as had two more of her friends on the drug. Although that was annoying to a fashion-conscious lady like Valerie, she felt it was a small price to pay for having her life and both her breasts intact. She would live with the extra weight and work on losing it when she had finished the five-year course of Tamoxifen.

Valerie also said her immune system was shot after just radiotherapy, and that she picked up infections really easily. At the time she was recovering from the 'Marbella flu', poor thing.

In the evening we visited Pat's friends Jocelyn and Ciaran. Like Pat, Jocelyn is a wonderful cook and I ate three helpings of delicious paella without upsetting my digestion. Medically trained and very knowledgeable, Jocelyn is the practice manager for Mr Adriaan Grobbelaar, a consultant plastic surgeon who specialises in palsy and reconstruction, including breast. She said that I would conquer my cancer because I was strong. Sometimes I don't feel strong at all but I think that having people believe in you spurs you on.

Jocelyn kindly examined my left arm, still swollen and painful (both lower and upper) several weeks after it was bruised when cannulated for the second time during my second chemo. I was worried about it and wondered if it might have become infected but Jocelyn said it would feel hot if infected and it was not. But it was to get worse...

WEDNESDAY 3RD OCTOBER:
The Inspiration Awards For Women

I returned from Marbella feeling so much better after some healing sun and sea (the weather had turned hot again after two damp days.) That evening my friend, PR extraordinaire Pammie Sharrock, had invited me to present an award at the prestigious Inspiration Awards For Women, in aid of Breakthrough Breast Cancer during Breast Cancer Awareness Month and sponsored by Lovelite, which she was helping to organise with Stella Brockway. It was a wonderful event anchored by Andrew Castle and Donna Air and the other presenters included Brendan Cole, Jo Wood and Ingrid Tarrant. The award I presented was won by the truly inspirational Aung San Suu Kyi who was sadly in Burma, so I nearly got to go home with it myself!

I took Jade and enjoyed seeing old friends. Sweet Ingrid kindly bought me a lovely little heart 'pod' designed by Charlotte Biehl, who had generously donated the presenters' bracelets for the event. Healthy Ingrid dropped us home afterwards and gave me lots of useful nutritional advice.

THURSDAY 4TH OCTOBER:
My Left Arm, Part One

My whole left arm has been painful and stiff after swelling up again in Spain and I had to take painkillers to control the pain. The chemist did not want to give me anything without my seeing my doctors, so I trotted off to the Marsden once again and saw Dr Tazia at the MDU. She said that the bruised, cannulated vein was very inflamed and prescribed Voltarol gel and an antibiotic called Flucloxacillin to prevent a possible blood clot. Oh no – just when I thought it was safe to go back in the water and get off the antibiotics! My poor vein.

Dr Tazia said that the corresponding large back vein in the right arm had softened and should be useable next time, even though it felt a bit sore. But did I want to run the risk of having the same thing happen to my right arm? Had the vein swelled up because it had been cannulated twice? If I could only use each arm vein once not twice, I was running out of veins!

I discussed the possibility of having a permanent PICC line inserted into my upper arm to save my veins but when reading the information about it in the leaflet Dr Tazia gave me, I discovered that the line would run right up to my heart and that it required a plastic sleeve for showering. It all sounded a bit grim.

I was upset that my vein swelled up again after it had settled down and wondered if I could have inadvertently knocked it when I exfoliated my skin in Spain last Sunday. I realise now that you cannot do everything you normally do whilst on chemo. You have to accept you are much more fragile than usual and treat yourself with kid gloves. When my arm finally heals I think I will put a wee bandage on it to remind me to be extra careful about touching it. When it first swelled up one of my doctors *had* told me that it would take a few months to settle down.

FRIDAY 5TH OCTOBER:
Macmillan Coffee Morning

This morning I attended Sir Paul Judge's Champagne and Coffee Morning in aid of Macmillan's, for Breast Cancer Awareness Month. I bought a healthy and delicious wheat-and-dairy-free cake made by a jolly girl called Poppy and had a fun time in spite of my arm. Paul's co-host Suki had suffered from breast cancer two years ago but was now very healthy, cheerful and upbeat.

SATURDAY 6TH OCTOBER:
My Left Arm, Part Two

Today I was in panic mode about my painful arm and emailed everyone I knew who had had chemo, to ask for advice. All of them said they had had vein problems and had had Ports put in which were brilliant. Thank God it is not just me with this vein problem.

I read up about the 'Portacath' in the leaflet and decided it would be much safer than the PICC line as it would be secured under my skin. (A Portacath is a small medical appliance installed beneath the skin and a catheter connects the Port to a vein.) However the PICC line can be put in at the MDU before chemo whereas the Port requires a little operation, an anaesthetic and a scar. Health must rule over beauty – I need my veins to transport my blood!

Being so squeamish, I am blooming terrified of both of these things; I don't know which would be worse – having the PICC put in with<u>out</u> an anaesthetic or having a much feared anaesthetic for the Port. I do not like the thought of having any foreign body put inside me but desperate situations call for desperate measures. My poor veins are unhappy, I am in pain and having to take painkillers which then exacerbate my stomach acidity. I need to take action.

SUNDAY 7TH OCTOBER:
Tales Of Hecuba

After a couple of rehearsals, Jade and I appeared in a play reading for Jackie Skarvellis's new play *Tales Of Hecuba* at Theatro Technis today. Jackie had invited some producers in the hope of getting the play put on in the West End and had gathered a good team of actors together. I played Helen Of Troy, Jade was Polyxena and happily the play was very well received. I thoroughly enjoyed playing naughty Helen – with the only funny lines in the tragedy I was really able to camp it up! And Jade was wonderful as the doomed Polyxena who gets executed by firing squad. I think I should take a leaf out of Helen's book and become a Strong Woman – I cannot imagine The Face That Launched A Thousand Ships wincing and whingeing over a spot of pain!

Afterwards we had dinner with our friends Dominic (Lord) Mereworth, Walter Bamford, Vivien King-Lawless and Valerie Austin, and I wolfed down a moussaka with no ill-effects. My arm was still painful even after four days of antibiotics but I find that regular Paracetamol and the Voltarol gel help.

MONDAY 8TH OCTOBER:
Anna Karenina

My arm was slightly better today on the fifth day of antibiotics and I sat through two hours of a BAFTA screening of
the new and artistic version of *Anna Karenina* plus a
fascinating but lengthy Q&A with Keira Knightley and
director Joe Wright without having to take any painkillers.

TUESDAY 9TH OCTOBER:
Sir Roger And A Porsche

My arm has not yet healed, although it is getting less
painful and I have been rather bad tempered – either from
the Paracetamol or the Flucloxacillin or both. I enjoyed a
Roger Moore book-signing evening with my good friends
Tatiana and Kenteas but am having to drive one-handed at
the moment and unfortunately reversed into a rather nice
Porsche on my street! Luckily no harm was done but I have
decided to ditch the car until my left arm is working again.

WEDNESDAY 10TH OCTOBER:
The Prof's Advice, A Tank And A Fashion Show

I wobbled off to the Marsden one-handed on my bike,
feeling very depressed and weepy about my vein situation.
This is the worst thing that has happened to me during
chemo – even worse than the scary bleeding, because that

stopped quickly and this has gone on for so long. However, various members of my oncological team – the wonderful Professor Smith, his cheerful PA Geraldine and the sweet Dr G Anandappa – were all there today and soon managed to cheer me up.

The Prof said that he would get on to my surgeon, Mr Gui, about having a Port put in asap but suggested I try to have the usual IV chemo tomorrow – if none of my veins are in working order, I will just have to go home again. He told me that Taxol was an easier drug to administer intravenously than EC, and won't irritate the veins so much. He also said that, on the whole, the side-effects were less bad with Taxol although I might now get some tingling and numbness in my hands and feet. One of the things I like about Professor Smith is that he is very honest, and he told me that I might get some pain in the bones, especially my back, on Taxol but that I could control this with painkillers.

Later I told my lawyer pal Mike Cooper about my latest problem and he said I was 'like a tank' – things kept blowing up but I just shifted down into first gear and kept ploughing ahead! I responded that he too was like a tank with my case against News International, which he is handling for me – the 'Operation Wheating' police had warned me that I had been hacked by the News of The World and I had joined the class action to sue the company. What's good enough for Jude Law, Sienna Miller and Hugh Grant is good enough for me!

Feeling happier, I attended Rachel Couture's glitzy fashion show organised by my pal and PR Charlotte at the Millennium Chelsea Hotel with Princess Katarina and Denise and Chantelle Pidgley. I loved ogling the pretty frocks and was pleased when Prince Mohsin Ali Khan offered to send me some remote healing. It is amazing how many people are into healing these days – if it did not work they would not all be doing it. I hope it works on my poor arm.

THURSDAY 11TH OCTOBER:
5th Chemo / 1st Taxol

My ultrasound with Dr Allen revealed that my tumours are now no bigger than 1.3 centimetres – yay! All the pain and anxiety are worth it.

I bumped into sympathetic nurse Orla whom I had not seen for a while and she warned me that implanting a Port is surgery and involves a general anaesthetic and that I should only have it if I really had exhausted all my vein options – oh gawd!

Then it was chemo time with the new drug, Accelerated Paclitaxel. The Prof had requested the most experienced cannulation nurse for me and I was delighted with charming Australian senior staff nurse Sophie – when she put the needle in, it really was just a tiny scratch. With the help of another nice nurse, Jeannette, and Jade's support, Sophie kept me as comfortable as possible. She found a new 'good' vein on the side of my left arm that did not touch my damaged vein at all.

Firstly Sophie flushed, then administered the pre-meds – steroids for nausea and Piriton for allergies – which made me quite dozy during the three hours of Taxol. I watched *Desperate Housewives* on the hospital computer with headphones purchased by Jade from the hospital shop but do not remember much of the plot!

Then more flushing and I was finished. As before, I had my Lorazepam and anaesthetic gel half an hour before treatment and it wasn't too bad – a bit of discomfort while the pre-meds went in but the actual Taxol was administered so slowly that I hardly felt a thing.

I had given up the ice cap as it would have meant wearing it for four hours and I would not have been able to tolerate it. I have got used to wearing baseball caps and my Crystal wig now. Everybody admires Crystal enormously – the Prof asked to touch it yesterday and pronounced it very realistic.

Sophie is a very knowledgeable nurse and informed me that I was able to have massage whilst undergoing chemo: it is a myth that massaging spreads cancer cells. (There are so many myths about cancer and chemo but I am gradually getting to the bottom of it all.)

She also explained about the rectal bleeding I had had last time, which had freaked me out so much. She said that the scary, free-flowing bleeding could have been due to low platelets (platelets help blood to clot) and that I should be careful this time as well (nappy time, I wondered? Gross!).

I also mentioned that, although I had only put on a few pounds in spite of all the food I had been eating (the steroids make you hungry), I had actually 'spread' quite a lot around my tummy and waist area and could not now fit into some of my favourite clothes. I had noticed this when wriggling into various outfits for Rachel's fashion show and eventually plumping (excuse the pun) for a stretchy dress that did not make me look like a sausage or show off my new pot belly! Sophie said it was quite normal to change body shape during chemo and that I would go back to my usual size afterwards.

Robert, my regular driver, said he liked me looking a bit bigger 'without little stick legs'. Forget the stick legs, it is the pot belly I am not appreciating!

While in the MDU today, Jade and I noticed a poor lady who was there for the first time by herself and in floods of tears. She was obviously very frightened, as I had been the first time – fear of the unknown mainly.

ADVICE: If you can, always take a friend or family member with you for chemo (and any hospital visit when you might be anxious) to hold your hand and take your mind off things.

This nice lady said that she had not wanted to put any of her friends or family through the chemo experience. God bless her kindness. She perked up later once she realised, as we all do, that the treatment is not too bad and the Marsden nurses are all so good. She said she was having eight chemos for cancer of the lymph and was hoping to carry on her work in a school. With our four sessions' worth of experience as chemo buddy and patient, Jade and I were able to advise her not to overdo it and to rest a lot when not working but that all the side-effects were manageable with the right medicines.

I went home feeling quite woozy and collapsed in front of *Strictly Come Dancing*. But I was also pleased: we had found a vein and I had got through the session rather than being sent home, which would have made me feel a failure.

After a week, the Flucloxacillin had worked and my bruised vein was more comfortable and I could use my arm without pain once again – hooray!

SATURDAY 13TH OCTOBER:
Back To Massage

I did not want to jinx it but I was feeling much better this time. I had been sent home with just one anti-nausea drug, the Domperidone, and I had not had the usual nausea and acidity, was sleeping reasonably well without pills and just had a mild flush (not unattractive actually!) for the first day or so. So I decided to take Sophie's advice and have a nice massage at my beauty therapist, Kamini Beauty in Kensington. Kami's massage therapist Yukie specialises in deep tissue massage and Swedish massage but I decided to have a relaxing massage instead today, as I am quite fragile at the moment. Yukie avoided the veins in my arms and gave me a lovely gentle massage, which sent me to sleep. It was blissful and I decided to treat myself regularly now I knew it was 'allowed.'

TUESDAY 16TH OCTOBER:
Taxol Side-Effects – And Billy, Geoff, Heather And Sir Francis

For the last few days I have monitored myself after my first Taxol. The first three days I felt much better than usual with no horrid nausea, acidity, insomnia and other side-effects. Since Sunday, though, I've felt a bit ache-y in my bones and muscles, which I understand is normal, and the district nurse has come round to give me an injection three days running to control this. My stomach has also been a bit uncomfortable and swollen from time to time. I did not take any painkillers in case they brought on the usual beastly acidity but, if this is as bad as it gets, I can handle it.

Today dear old Billy Carter rang. He is such a trouper. The doctors have now told him he has only got 'til May to live and he has developed a horrid side-effect of producing too much saliva, so he wakes up every day with a pool of it on his pillow. But his spirit is indomitable; he is taking soursop, the wonder, cancer-killing fruit from Brazil, and he is fighting on bravely, although coughing a lot, poor thing.

As always, Billy told me some uplifting cancer stories. One was about a man he knows who had a brain tumour and was given one month to live five years ago. He received treatment from the private Dove Clinic in Harley Street and is still with us, having regular blood transfusions every month to get rid of cancerous blood and deliver 'clean' blood. Apparently this costs about £1,000 a time at the clinic.

I remember when one of my dearest platonic men friends, the Charles Dickens actor Geoffrey 'Nanny Geoff' Harris, was suffering from multiple cancers he used to have regular blood transfusions and they perked him up no end. Geoff was a wonderful chap who looked after Jade when she was young and we never believed he would actually die. In those days I didn't know much about cancer and I thought because my friend Ann-Marie survived, all my friends with cancer would live. When Geoff died, Jade and I were devastated and we still miss him. Jade's lovely agent Heather had got breast cancer when only thirty-three and died of liver cancer when only thirty-eight – such a tragedy. God rest their souls.

That is when I realised that you are more likely to die if

your cancer 'metastasises', i.e. travels to another area of the body (although the sterling Prudence – the extraordinary lady who wrote to me when I was working at the Drayton Theatre – is living with five cancers, God bless her.) Let's hope dear Billy will be the male Prudence. In any case, Billy is living a very healthy life. He walks two miles in the fresh country air every day and reminded me of the story of Sir Francis Chichester, the famous yachtsman. Apparently Sir Francis was diagnosed with cancer and given one month to live. He bravely chose to sail around the world on his boat Gypsy Moth for four-and-a-half years and the exercise of manning the sails and the fresh sea air kept him going. Sadly he died one month after returning to a normal life.

WEDNESDAY 17TH OCTOBER:
To Port Or Not To Port, That Is The Question

I went to see Mr Gui with nurse Orla, feeling depressed over the possibility of having to have a Port inserted, and he kindly said he had heard I had been triumphing over my tumours 'like a Trojan'. This cheered me up and made me laugh; having just played Helen Of Troy at Jackie Skarvellis's recent play reading I definitely think Trojan! Mr Gui said he would support me if I really wanted the Port but that it would involve surgery, there was a risk of infection and of affecting the lungs. There would also be a permanent scar and from the look of my skin in the area, I would not scar well, he said. Was it really worth it for just three more cannulations?

I took all these things on board plus the fact that, as

Professor Smith had told me, the Taxol had not irritated the vein nurse Sophie had cannulated in the way EC had done. Mr Gui examined my veins and said the sore, cannulated ones should settle down in time and that he reckoned there were enough other good veins for Sophie to use for the last three chemos. We left it that he would speak to Sophie about my veins and hope that she would be confident that she could get me through the next three sessions.

Then he examined the tumour area, seemed pleased and we discussed possible dates for the surgery. If my blood count is good enough each time for the last three chemos, and I finish on time on the 22nd November, he could safely operate on the 13th December. Then I would have Christmas to recuperate and six weeks later start the month's course of radiotherapy. So hopefully I will be finished with everything and able to go skiing and start my next play by March 2013!

If there are any problems, the next surgery date will be 27th December. I am to have a pre-op assessment on the 5th December.

I left the Marsden feeling much happier – the end is in sight! Mr Gui always fills me with confidence; he really knows his stuff and I am so lucky he is my surgeon.

THURSDAY 18TH OCTOBER:
Getting Sparkly!

In general I am feeling much better on Taxol. The only thing I've noticed is that my stomach gets a bit painful and swollen from time to time and I have to be very careful what I eat, with nothing spicy whatsoever (although this might just be a cumulative effect of chemo in general.)

I noticed this today when Vivien took me off to her latest couture contact, Medici in Margaret Street, to borrow a dress for the upcoming James Bond premiere, *Skyfall*, which Charlotte had cleverly got tickets for. Jeremy and I had bought Jade a slinky dress and her first Manolo Blahnik shoes for her 21st birthday at the end of the month and I wanted to keep up with her! Between Jade, Viv and the manager Andrea, we found a gorgeous silver sparkly dress which was draped just enough to conceal my current stomach imperfections!

Then Viv took me off to Nails Inc in Harvey Nichols, where manager Lauren painted silver sparkles on my nails to match my dress, with pink sparkles on my pinkies for Breast Cancer Awareness Month. I had noticed that my nails and toenails had become very weak and flaky on chemo and Lauren, an experienced nail technician, advised me to ditch my previous nail extension method of machine filing and acrylic and go for the gentler hand filing and gel. At least my nails haven't fallen off like some poor chemo patients. You have to be prepared for everything.

TUESDAY 23RD OCTOBER:
The Skyfall Premiere

The *Skyfall* premiere was an historic event, the biggest and best Royal film premiere this country has ever seen. The whole of the back of the Royal Albert Hall was turned into one gigantic red carpet area where the fans could admire all the Bond Boys and Girls as well as The Prince of Wales and The Duchess of Cornwall.

My cancer mate Billy, who had taken the stills on several Bond movies, came up from Suffolk with his wife and carer Harumi, and his friend Ken donned a chauffeur's cap and drove us all in his vintage red Rolls Royce. Jade's good friend Chantelle came along and we met my pal Raj who was also chauffered up in a vintage car – all very James Bond!

Billy was looking amazingly well considering what he has been through with his three cancers. His famous mane of silver hair has grown back thicker and his face looks very young (I believe the chemo steroids swell the face slightly and make people look younger – there have to be some advantages to such an unpleasant treatment, even if only superficial).

We all had a wonderful time poncing about on the red carpet, rubbing shoulders with gorgeous 007 Daniel Craig, signing autographs and grinning for the snappers. I think the high point of my career was one of the photographs later published on the Internet where Jade, Chantelle and I were in the foreground and the divine Ralph Fiennes was in the background!

It was great to see Billy enjoying himself so much and attending such an amazing event, and seeing so many friends also cheered me up a lot. Billy was sporting two badges saying 'Cancer Sucks' – that is certainly true but it makes you appreciate the fun times more.

The film was brilliant, one of the best-ever Bonds, and I was pleased that my veins had settled down so that I did not have to worry too much about them being knocked in the huge crowd at the Albert Hall.

WEDNESDAY 24TH OCTOBER:
My Vein Conditions And Elena On Nutrition

Back to reality! I saw Professor Smith and said how pleased I was that I had not in fact had a Port inserted because the Taxol cannulation did not seem to have irritated my vein at all. I learnt that the condition I had had on my left large vein was 'thrombophlebitis' whereas what had happened to my right large vein that prevented any more cannulation was just 'sclerosis' (hardening).

Regarding my Taxol side-effects, I reported that I could tolerate the slight tingling and aches and that I was being careful about my stomach. The Prof thought everything was normal. Then I had a long chat with senior staff nurse Elena, whose opinion I also value, about nutrition. Elena said that there is no medical or scientific proof that following the Cancer Diet to the letter helps kill cancer and that instances of people apparently curing themselves by eating just raw fruit and veg could be coincidental. You should just aim to 'eat well' all the time, she said. She also said that Iscador, made from mistletoe extracts, is being used as a cancer medicine, whereas she had not heard of Billy's soursop, the Brazilian fruit. I know the medics can only tell you what is actually medically proven and it's good to hear that they have embraced Iscador, made from a plant. My feeling is to stick to the Diet as well as having my medical treatment – it cannot do any harm and *may* do some good! But at least after talking to the sensible Elena I am not going to obsess about it.

THURSDAY 25TH OCTOBER:
6th Chemo / 2nd Taxol

Today was a bit like a cocktail party round my chair at the MDU! Firstly Jacquie Gulbenkian, Vivien's friend who helps run The Friends Of The Royal Marsden, popped along to say 'hi' to me and asked me to pose with a gorgeous Lulu Guinness tote bag which was being sold in aid of The Friends. I was delighted to follow in the footsteps of Joan Collins and Robert Lindsay, who had also posed for the cause, and was so busy preening with the bag that I hardly noticed the wonderful nurse Sophie inserting the dreaded cannula. I had put some lipstick on to be 'ready for my close up, Mr DeMille' and Dr Tazia remarked that I was looking very pretty today – the wonders of modern make-up!

Then my childhood friend Biffa Ogier, whom I had not seen for ages, arrived. It turns out she is also a Friends volunteer and Jacquie had told her I was there. It was great to meet Jacquie and see Biffa and it really took my mind off the cannulation, which was a bit uncomfortable today in my small right vein. It felt better when nurse Kathryn wrapped a heat pad round it to open up the vein a bit. I remembered that I had had my arm dipped in hot water before putting the drugs in the previous time. The anaesthetic gel I always have put on half an hour before the injection shrinks the vein, making it smaller and less comfortable for the drugs to pass through – but I wouldn't give up my anaesthetic, I am too much of a wimp! Therefore I need some heat to open up the vein again.

ADVICE: *If you are having a smaller vein cannulated, whether or not you have the anaesthetic gel (which I recommend if you are needle phobic) and your stomach acidity levels can take it, take a couple of Paracetamol before cannulation.*

Apparently the pre-meds before the actual Taxol are worse than the drug itself but I found it all a bit uncomfortable today. Pain is stressful and must be avoided unless absolutely necessary. I was very lucky that nurses Sophie and Kathryn are so gentle. However I managed to shoot myself in the foot at the end of my treatment by running to the loo with my cannula still in and – of course – knocking it out by mistake, plonker that I am! As I watched the blood bloom like a carnation onto the white pad I felt instantly nauseous and weak as a kitten and realised that, although I am generally much less needle phobic, I have not got over my blood phobia and must have another hypno session with Lucien asap.

Kathyrn staunched the bleeding immediately but I have learned my lesson and will cross my legs next time and let the nurse take the cannula out *before* going to the loo.

SUNDAY 28TH OCTOBER:
Taxol Side-Effects

My side-effects this time are just like last time – a bit of insomnia, a mild flush, a tiny bit of tingling in the fingertips and the aches and pains start on the third day, i.e. today. But this time I also had a nosebleed, which means it is official: I have now had every chemo side-effect mentioned in the hospital flyer except vomiting, not to mention one they do not mention!

MONDAY 29TH OCTOBER:
District Nurse Mary, Lucien, Jack And Bernie

I dosed myself up with Paracetamol for the aches and pains and 'vein ache' and Lanzoprazole for the acidity from the painkillers, and staggered through my 'Ladies' Matchplay' tennis coaching with a jolly bunch of ladies at Hurlingham with lots of sit downs! Having no energy to run has actually made me become more accurate with my shots – interesting.

Lucien came over to give me hypno for my blood phobia and healing for my veins. I do not know how these things work, they just seem to: after treatment my veins immediately felt less ache-y. Mind over matter, I guess.

All the district nurses who have come over to give me my shots after the chemo treatments have been delightful but tonight I think I shocked the latest one, nurse Mary. I was going out later so was all tarted up when I opened the door.

Mary said, 'Where's Sally?'

I said, 'I'm Sally'.

'No', she said, 'you are not a cancer patient!'

Jade and I smiled and explained the wonders of the NHS wiggly, Jinny lashes and loads of blusher (I look like a waxwork without make-up). I just know that if you look good, you feel good.

There was sad news today. My agent Michele Hart rang me to say that 'Black' Jack Dellal had died. He was a long-time boyfriend of mine in the eighties, a very kind and generous man. He was eighty-nine years old and had had a fabulous life, embodying the spirit of 'live each day'. Goodbye to Jack, a colourful character.

Then I read in the paper that Bernie Nolan, 52, the Irish singer who had whipped breast cancer previously, was ill again. The cancer had returned to her brain, lungs, liver and bones but she vowed to fight it, saying, 'It's not curable. I'm on medication, which is controlling it, and people have lived for twelve years on these drugs. Who knows what new treatments are round the corner?'

Bernie is so right, the medics are finding new treatments all the time. What an incredibly brave and inspiring lady. It makes you wonder if you could be so strong yourself if it happened to you. Courageous Bernie has a young daughter and she will stay strong for her girl. I said a little prayer for her and everybody who I know and do not know who is fighting this beastly, deadly disease.

SUNDAY 4th NOVEMBER:
Jade's 21st, Parties And 'Go With The Flow'

This week was my Jade's twenty-first birthday! I felt a bit guilty because I had wanted to throw her a huge jamboree at Longleat. She said she did not want a big do, but I knew it was because she did not want me to have the stress of organising it in my current debilitated state, bless her.

In the event she dined and clubbed with her five close girlfriends, Minnie, Milla, Hannah, India and Savannah, on Wednesday and they and other friends and Allie organised a wonderful party for her at Minnie's house in Leeds, where many of her pals are studying, at the weekend. They all had a brilliant time and Jade said it was the best party ever – and no stress for mumma!

As it happened I am feeling OK at the moment – tired most of the time but my veins are more comfortable and I actually managed to attend the glitzy openings of Buddha Bar and Mash in sleeveless frocks this week without worrying about knocking my arms. The only new problem I have is some itchy little 'blood blemishes' on my arms and hands but I will talk to the doctors about them this week.

Nothing surprises me on the side-effects front any more. I am still feeling bloated and can't get some of my rings and size eight clothes on – although Adele has kindly given me some of her size tens to tide me over. But, as Jade said, at least I haven't gone the other way and become really skinny. Some of the chemo patients we have seen have been so heartbreakingly skeletal. I know it upsets Jade a lot because she is a compassionate creature and I am so grateful for her company at the hospital every time but some of the patients we see in their wheelchairs look so frail and we can only hope and pray that they will make it.

I still have regular insomnia but use the time to read lots of books, the latest being the excellent cancer book *Go With The Flow*, by acclaimed photographer Gemma Levine. Gemma got breast cancer at a mature age but whipped it after having a mastectomy, chemo and radiotherapy. She has used her cancer experience to create a wonderful book where the practitioners, researchers, support staff and therapists who treated her on her journey have shared their valuable knowledge. There are comprehensive chapters by the experts on not just the actual surgery, chemo and radio but also remedial massage, dentistry, podiatry, post-mastectomy bra fittings and make-up, and Gemma has added her own special exercises for mastectomy patients. She has also included her trademark photographs of each expert and quotes about cancer from celebrity friends such as Dame Joan Bakewell, Dame Kiri Te Kanawa, Angela Rippon, David Suchet, Joanna Lumley and Gloria Hunniford, who makes the important point that her gorgeous daughter Caron Keating tragically died before the current lifesaving cancer drugs had been released on the market.

Interestingly, Gemma is one of only two people I have heard of who did *not* lose their hair. She used the ice cap and includes a whole chapter about exactly how the cap works and its history. Very encouraging – and her silver mane certainly looks wonderful on the cover of the book.

Gemma generously donates all the royalties from her book to Maggie's Cancer Caring Centres. The quote at the end of the book from her son James says it all: Mum 1; Cancer 0. I hope and pray that this will be the case with more and more patients in the future as, with valuable research, the treatments improve all the time.

MONDAY 5TH NOVEMBER:
Flu Shot

I had my annual 'flu shot. You are allowed these whilst on chemo and it is a good idea as, if you contracted some horrid strain of 'flu you might run a high temperature and have to be admitted to hospital. I felt a bit fluey within the next 24 hours but that was all.

WEDNESDAY 7TH NOVEMBER:
Big In Size And Big In Spain?

Today at the Marsden I saw a very smart lady doctor called Dr Amna Sheri. She told me that the funny little red marks on my arms were most likely chemo side-effects, that my painful right vein was just sclerosis, not more thrombophebitis (thank God!) and that the uncomfortable swelling and fluid retention I was experiencing was quite normal and would go down a few weeks after 'chemo's end'. What a relief – I had been very upset recently when dressing for a 'do' and discovering that I could not manage to stuff my grandmother's gorgeous pearl and diamond ring onto my now porky little finger! That ring had been lost for months in the bottom of my model bag, been retrieved from a drain in Disneyland and had its pearl re-stuck on by Ozzi Friedlander, my jeweller, but somehow always came back to me. I am dying to wear it again.

I asked Dr Sheri if my current three-in-a-row daily boosters with the district nurse were for the aches and pains of Taxol or for my immune system, as with the big booster I used to have the day after my EC. The doctor explained that the big booster shot could exacerbate aches and pains, which is why they gave the three smaller shots after Taxol (which can also give you aches and pains) but that they were in fact for the immune system. Well, they have worked up till now. In fact I read the leaflet about the Zarzio booster injections and noticed that one of the common side-effects was a 'rash', so maybe that is what my itchy little red marks are.

After my consultation, I had a job. My cousin Nick Broom

had kindly recommended me to TVE, the Spanish BBC, to do an etiquette show on ladies who lunch. I had not done an etiquette show since presenting *How To Marry A Million-aire* ten years ago (and, thinking about it, that could have been more about gold-digging than etiquette!).

Never mind, I needed the money so I brushed up on my etiquette skills and stuffed myself into one of the few suits I could still get into. As I struggled with the zip, I was reminded of watching a telly show about Liberace when I was young. The great entertainer was showing off his wardrobe and revealed that he had 'thin clothes, fat clothes and in-between clothes', for the various stages of his various diets. This is clearly what you need if you put on or take off weight whilst on chemo. I only noticed my weight gain about halfway through my chemo course; I have put on about half a stone in weight, one seventeenth of my entire body weight and one dress size, which is about two inches all over. For us ladies, one dress size makes all the differ-ence and I am having to have a good rootle around in the old wardrobe these days.

Once in the suit, I raced off to the Millennium Mayfair Hotel where my PR pal Annie McKale was letting us film. My friends Charlotte, Vivien and Iris Bond, were my fellow lunching ladies and we had a great time and the shoot went really well. Nick Easen, the producer, was delightful and I do not think they guessed for one moment that I was ill. I would have difficulty getting a long telly job or theatre run at the moment, due to the insurance producers need for artistes, so I'm grateful for anything. Maybe the ladies and I will become 'big in Spain' – hopefully not in dress size!

THURSDAY 8TH NOVEMBER:
7th / Penultimate Chemo

When I turned up at the MDU today I was devastated to hear that the wonderful senior nurse Sophie was off today. I requested 'the best senior nurse available, please', explaining about my thrombophlebitis, sclerosis and general dodgy state of my veins, not to mention my IV phobia but was told one usually had to take pot luck. Being a polite little British person and not wishing to steal a nurse away from other deserving patients, I said 'OK'. Bad mistake! I should have used my acting skills and had a nervous breakdown or asked to wait as long as it took to get a senior nurse.

In the event two sweet junior nurses tried unsuccessfully to cannulate my veins and nearly had nervous breakdowns themselves! The first nurse said she had done it before and 'thought she could do it' but could not get the cannula into my right small vein (cannulated successfully last time but perhaps it was too early to try it again) and broke down in tears because she had obviously hurt me quite a lot. Oh no – then I had guilt on my shoulders as well as pain in my arm!

The second junior nurse had a go at two of the smaller front veins on my left arm, my large back vein still not having recovered from the thrombophlebitis. It really hurt and I am ashamed to say that I then burst into tears, followed closely by poor Jade who was devastated to see her mumma in pain. I always try to keep it together in front of my child but this was a truly horrid moment. I had been given the tranquiliser, painkillers and the anaesthetic patches on my veins but nothing helped – it was just too blooming nasty for fraidy cat moi – and I was getting quite upset, saying, 'I am not a guinea pig, I am not a pin cushion!'

I was trying to do my relaxing deep breathing but was in fact hyperventilating with anxiety. The nurse said she would have to take the (third) cannula out but I was begging her to please leave it in and push harder. It was a real 'Samantha' in *Sex And The City* moment! I said, 'I have been through childbirth and Botox, I can take the pain, I <u>have</u> to get through this chemo today and the next one in two weeks' time so that I can keep my surgery date and get on with my life.' But the cannula just would not go in properly so she had to remove it and I collapsed in a snivelling heap. When I asked the first nurse where the second nurse had gone, she said, 'Oh, she has left the country!'

Finally a lovely senior nurse called Sally (a good omen) appeared, immersed my arm in a bucket of very hot water, then immediately cannulated my outer big vein quickly, safely and comfortably. Now why didn't I think of that clever wheeze? It must be very demoralising for the whole unit when both patients and staff are in tears!

I quite understand that they have lots of sick patients to deal with but some have Picc Lines and Ports and I envied those ones today. I guess patients like me who are near the end of their course, when the veins are at their worst, need to be really careful. Still, I am lucky I am at the Marsden, where all the nurses are so gentle and caring and I felt so sorry that the poor nurses had felt so bad for me.

Once cannulated by Sally, the first nurse, who had by now recovered luckily, took over to administer the drugs. I finally felt the famous 'prickly hedgehog' that nurse Beth had told me about when the nurse put the pre-meds in. I did not just feel as if I was <u>sitting</u> on a prickly hedgehog but as if I had prickly hedgehogs running all over me! It did not feel painful, just a bit uncomfortable and funny. The nurse immediately slowed down the drug and the feeling went off. I think I am a person who needs my drugs administered really slowly for some reason.

The rest was plain sailing and comfortable in the big back vein. I occasionally felt a twinge round the cannulation area but finally passed out with the thrill of it all – or it could have been the combination of the tranquiliser and the Piriton pre-med! Apparently Jacquie Gulbenkian from The Friends Of The Marsden came round to see me but said I was sleeping and looked 'beautiful and peaceful' – knackered, I reckon.

Later on, my long-time friend and Jade's Godmum, Patricia Madden, popped in to see me, bringing me very welcome ginger ale and yoghurt and kept Jade and me amused with stories of the hols we had gone on together to Israel when I was pregnant with Jade and tales of her fiancé and her menagerie, not necessarily in that order. Patricia's wit and good spirits cheered me up a lot but when I got home I had to have a huge glass of wine – now red for health reasons – to get over my cannula ordeal! I was feeling very sorry for myself and rang up fellow cancer sufferer Billy Carter to have a moan. Billy put things into perspective by telling me that, at his fourth chemo, the nurses had tried to cannulate his veins nine times without success at the Royal Free, another excellent cancer hospital. Billy said he finally pulled the last cannula out, walked out of the unit and demanded to see the head of the hospital and have a Port put in immediately. That worked well for him and still does, now that he has Herceptin administered every month via the Port.

ADVICE: VEINS. *Before you start your chemo course take a good look at your veins and, if you think they are not very prominent (we are talking Madonna here!), enquire about a Picc Line, a Hickman Line and a Port. This is especially important if you are going to have a long course of chemo and maybe Herceptin intravenously afterwards.*

I have always thought I have prominent veins. In fact when I was modelling full time and using my hands for nail polish adverts, etc, I always had to put them in the air to make the blood run down from the veins and make my hands look smooth. But a cannula is a blooming big thing to get in and it is no fun when the nurse has to 'push' the drugs through a delicate front vein. Like Billy, my veins were already bruised and uncomfortable by the fourth chemo session. If you are having chemo every week, for instance, it does not give your veins time to recover.

It is a good idea to make a note of which veins have been cannulated and when, so that you can alternate and keep using the veins used less recently. The pain and anxiety of having complaining veins 'invaded' by a large cannula are stressful for anybody, especially vulnerable cancer patients, and those patients I know who had Ports inserted were all so grateful to then have completely painless drug administration. I do not know anybody who has had one of the 'lines' – you need to discuss what is best for you with the doctors <u>before</u> you start your course.

Many chemo patients I have spoken to recently have had

problems with their veins – pain, bruising, discomfort – but have thought 'oh, it is just me'. Well, it is not 'just you', it happens to most people and please make it easier on yourself and enquire about your options in good time. And immersing your arm in really hot water works as well as the anaesthetic gel but keeps the veins large rather than shrinking them.

When I got home I looked at the paper to read about how Obama had squeaked home to a second term in the US election. The front page screamed 'Surgeon Botched 1,000 Breast Ops' and I read with mounting horror how a surgeon in the North of England had performed lumpectomies on patients with benign tumours and unsafe 'cleavage sparing' mastectomies on patients who had then got the cancer back. Awful – those poor women. It certainly put things in perspective and I stopped feeling so sorry for myself over a small bit of pain and tears.

This dreadful business reminded me that it is always worth getting a second opinion – and a third – and a fourth – if necessary. This is such an important lesson I have learned, not just from my own current cancer experience but from other medical situations within my family. Second opinions could have saved those poor ladies in the paper from having unnecessary or unsafe operations.

FRIDAY 9TH NOVEMBER:
Anna's Birthday

Today was my friend Anna Brocklebank's birthday and I rang to warble down the phone at her. I told her about my latest drama and she generously said, 'But my dear, you have shown so much courage, carried yourself with such aplomb and held your head high with dignity and style'. She should have seen me, the snivelling wreck, yesterday! But it is wonderful friends like Anna and their belief in me that keep me going and keep me strong. Today I just have a slightly sore vein, the usual slight flush and bags of energy from the steroids; plus I have regained my sense of humour.

TUESDAY 13TH NOVEMBER:
A Virus, Look Good...Feel Better And A Steak!

I have had my first bad cold and cough virus since being on chemo. It was brewing before I had both my 'flu shot and my last dose of chemo and could have been exacerbated by the muck sweat I got myself into at that last session. I have been super careful, staying in bed or at least indoors, keeping warm and taking my temperature regularly. The district nurse has been coming round to give me my boosters and I hope those will help.

After a couple of days, I got the usual mild aches and pains from chemo, and my energy levels hit the floor – I am as weak as a kitten.

I did not take my sleeping pills this time as I was on Benylin Original (great stuff) but have had my usual anxiety dreams of having hairy armpits, losing my handbag and not having my make-up on – very feminine! My subconscious anxiety may be because, with only one more chemo to go, I have been very aware that I am in the final furlong and must not fall at the last fence. If I can just get through the next two weeks and the nurses can find a vein for my last chemo, then I can start building up my immune system again and getting healthy for surgery and after.

I forgot to take my anti-sickness pills this time but found I did not need them. It has got to be good to cut down on any unnecessary pills while being pumped full of chemo drugs. There are definitely far fewer side-effects with Taxol.

ADVICE: I had a paper cut on my finger which didn't heal for ages (quite normal on chemo apparently) and the district nurse advised me to treat it – and any other cuts at the moment – by cleaning it with TCP, wearing a plaster in the daytime and letting it heal naturally at night. (It still took about three weeks to get better. 'Don't panic, Mr Mainwaring', as they say on my dad's favourite TV show, Dad's Army – you will eventually get there.)

In the afternoon I went to an excellent Look Good... Feel Better workshop at the wonderful Haven. I had heard great things about these workshops which help cancer/chemo patients to make the best of themselves whilst suffering from hair, brow and lash loss, dry skin, sores, weight adjustments and red skin (something which luckily only affects me for a couple of days).

Jill, a lovely lady from LG...FB, and her colleagues talked twelve of us through skin-care regimes and make-up and then sent us home with a gorgeous bag of goodies spon-sored by various manufacturers. It is always good to get tips from the experts and I also learned a lot from some of the other ladies, all of whom were sporting shaved heads, scarves, hats, wigs or half re-grown hair. The lady sitting next to me, who was fifty-one, had been on chemo on and off for twenty years after it had gone from her breast to her lungs and bones. She had stoically endured all those side-effects over the years and only recently decided to have a Port. What a trouper! I felt so humbled after having whinged about my veins after just seven sessions.

ADVICE: *This lady said that her hair had fallen out patchily, like mine, but that she had not shaved it all off and sometimes had extensions put in the long bits to 'flap' over the bald patches and that, although the texture of her new hair was different at first, it eventually reverted to type. I had been dithering as to whether or not to shave my remaining short hair off as it does shed and also sticks to moisturiser and make-up and gets in my eyes. However I will now keep what little I have got. Jade has assured me that I have 'little pricks' growing back on some of my bald patches already, possibly due to my diligently rubbing in hair restorer every night.*

The lady opposite me revealed that she had vomited constantly at first on EC. I have always reckoned I have had all the chemo side-effects because 'nausea and vomiting' were lumped together on the fact sheet but I have never actually vomited, and for that I am profoundly grateful. Vomiting is such a truly horrid sensation and so bad for your insides. I think I would endure ten other more minor side-effects to avoid vomiting and I am going to stop complaining now!

Another lady showed us her PICC line. I am so glad I did not have one as the end of it where they administer the drugs, take blood and so on actually hangs out of your arm, although covered by a neat stretchy bandage. I think it would have been impractical for me with my tennis, bike riding, red carpet frocks and general clumsiness. However, if you do not play sports, etc, and are prepared to be very careful and protective of your arm, I can see that it would work really well and save your veins.

In the evening Charlotte and I went to Mash, a glamorous new restaurant in the West End on the site of the old Titanic Club, so you feel as if you are eating in an ocean liner. I had attended the glitzy opening as Mash is publicised by my pal Ivan Rosenschein and knew that it is known for its excellent steaks. I allow myself red meat once a week and tonight was the night, so I gorged myself on a delicious Paraguyan fillet steak and really enjoyed it. I was a veggie for years due to my love of animals but had been eating meat since marrying Jeremy and having to cook for a household and had got used to it. If I eventually have to give up red meat entirely to ward off more cancer then I will do so. After all, I have got used to substituting agave syrup for sugar, soy and almond milk for dairy, dark chocolate for milk choc, red wine for white and cutting down on the wheat big time. Let's face it, how many of us have eaten meat-flavoured tofu in a Chinese restaurant and thought it was the real thing? I tried a delicious red wine and found I am getting more and more used to red, which is supposed to be so good for one.

WEDNESDAY 14TH NOVEMBER:
The Twilight Premiere And The Hippodrome

As I had enjoyed the *Skyfall* premiere so much I was keen to go to *The Twilight Saga: Breaking Dawn – Part 2* premiere tonight but was not sure if I should chance making my cough and cold worse. In the end I wrapped my warm Bangladeshi pashmina over my slinky evening dress, stuffed woolly tights into my skyscraper heels and trotted off with Rose-Marie. Nowadays when film makers premiere their *oeuvres* in Leicester Square they use the whole square as a giant red carpet and open the film in three or four of the cinemas there, so it is a huge event. The fans had been camping out for days and you could hear the screams for miles. At the time of writing this, everyone – especially their loyal fans – was wondering whether R Patz and Kris Stew were back together or not.

Rose-Marie and I had a great time going to the party at the Hampshire Hotel, tottering up the red carpet and inspecting the gorgeous *Twilight* actors. We both agreed that Taylor Lautner looks better since he has got older – there have to be some advantages to ageing! The film was fun and I realised that Lucien's hypnotherapy for my blood phobia must have finally worked as I did not have to turn my face away once in the gory bits!

Afterwards we went to the newly redesigned and re-opened Hippodrome Casino, where we watched a fab cabaret and had a nose around. I had started my compering career at The Hippodrome in the Eighties when Peter Stringfellow was in charge and did not think it would be the same without the great showman but the new Hippo staff were all lovely and looked after us really well. All the yummy food on the menu was very tempting and I was a bit naughty eating fish and chips and duck spring rolls. I guess I will have to be stricter when I finally come off chemo and start eating for The Rest Of My Life. As at Mash, I tried a nice red wine and found it was fine with fish and duck (sorry, purists!).

FRIDAY 16TH NOVEMBER:
Celebration And Sadness

The family news was good this week: Jade had done a nice job for the nation's best-selling newspaper, the super soar-away *Sun*, Kat's school had created a new job especially for her when the old one ended and Allie had been booked for another cooking season in Verbier. So it was time to celebrate and we had a late birthday dinner for the two girls at Scalini, a lively Italian restaurant in South Ken.

Mario, the owner, was an old friend and kindly said I could bring our own 'cancer diet' cake, so Jade and I zoomed off to collect it from Poppy, the nice cake-maker I had bought a cake from at Sir Paul Judge's Macmillan coffee morning. Poppy had excelled herself with a healthy no-wheat, no-dairy, no-sugar cake, which was not only safe for me but also good for Jade who likes to keep her skin perfect for her work – and of course the cake is slimming for everyone! Poppy told me one of her relations who had always been a tad tricky had mellowed considerably since having cancer and become much kinder to all his family.

Happily he is now on the mend. Certainly all the fellow cancer sufferers I have met seem to be very nice and kind. I wonder if we have all done 'deals with God?'

The dinner party for twenty-one people at Scalini, kindly hosted by my dear husband, was a huge success. I managed to resist all the delicious creamy pastas and ate prawns with papaya, and grilled liver, which I have been told is good for me. I certainly had plenty of champagne which one doctor had said was good for me and lots of red wine which everyone says is good for everyone!

We served the cake with optional cream and it was a huge hit. I have realised that you really do not have to eat loads of creamy, wheaty and sugary things to satisfy your taste buds and your stomach... that is all in the past now (well, maybe except at The Hippodrome!).

The only terribly sad note to the evening was when my sister-in-law Caroline told me that her employee's aunt, who had 'sailed though' chemo, then collapsed on a train station, had passed away. She had been wonderful, working throughout chemo to earn a living for her family, such a good woman. May she rest in peace.

MONDAY 19TH NOVEMBER:
Back To Pigging Out!

I have been feeling much more like me this second week. My veins are a bit sore and I am tired but I have had very little stomach pain, even when being quite daring in my eating habits, so I have been able to go to some very posh, rich food type events! Jeremy and I attended The Butterfly

Ball, where I consumed two different types of meat (it was my 'meat' day) with no ill-effects. The ball was in aid of The Rhys Daniels Trust, set up by Barry and Carmen Daniels when they tragically lost their two tiny children, Charly and Rhys, to Batten's Disease. When I am in pain or discomfort I often think of the inspirational Barry and other parents who have lost their children. Their heartache and bravery make my minor ailments feel truly minor.

A few days later, Jade and I attended the inaugural dinner of the World Peace and Prosperity Foundation, organised by our genius friends, chess grandmaster Raymond Keene and mind mapper Tony Buzan. It was chaired by Prince Mohsin Ali Khan and held at the House of Lords. It was Jade's first time at the Lords and she was suitably impressed with the beautiful buildings. The food was an Indian buffet, which I would not previously have dared eat but I dived in with a piled plate and felt fine. (Funnily enough when I returned from the Lords and removed my wiggly, I noticed a little spider nestling in the golden mass – occupational hazard with wigglies, I guess. Are there cobwebs in the House? At least it was a money spider – is it a sign that money is to come? He was a sweet little spider and I put him on the mantelpiece in my bedroom. A few days later I got a little part in a film – hmmn!)

Then my hair stylist friend, Russell Nurding, came up to visit me from Cirencester with our mutual pal, actress Eva Gray, and that involved a garlic-laden lunch at Da Mario. Still no ill-effects, hooray! Russell is a keen philanthropist who generously puts on fashion shows in aid of charity and I have modelled and compered for him several times with Eva.

ADVICE: *Interestingly, Russell told me that one of his staff had happily survived breast cancer, working on her feet all day in his salon throughout chemo (what a trouper!) but getting quite burnt by the radiotherapy. She had successfully used 99.9% aloe vera gel on the reddened skin.*

TUESDAY 20TH NOVEMBER:
After-Chemo Supplements To Rebuild The Immune System

Today I had a consultation with Patricia Peat from Cancer Options to discuss Life After Chemo and what supplements to take to rebuild my immune system. Patricia said I should keep up the three that I have been allowed to take during the treatment – multi vitamins, flax seed oil and Norwegian cod liver oil (particularly good, as chemo inflames the body and fish oil helps with this).

She said that, from seven days after the end of the chemo course, I should reinstate the following (I had taken them last year when my immune system first showed signs of weakness):

* Magnesium (chemo depletes this)

* Vitamin C with zinc – to combat colds, etc, and also good for wound healing, so particularly helpful post surgery.

* Calcium and vitamin D – better than vitamin D alone, as it helps protect against osteoporosis. Vitamin D is vital for stopping the inflammatory process, is important during the winter when there is no sun and gives one a higher chance of surviving breast cancer. (Patricia later told me

there had been a scare about breast cancer patients taking calcium and advised me to just take Vitamin D3 without Calcium. It's always best to check current thinking if you can.)

* Co-enzyme Q10 – which helps the body produce energy.

Post surgery, Patricia recommended adding:

* Vitamin E, vitamin B6 for healing and Maitake Japanese mushroom, which stimulates the body's natural killer cells.

Patricia said that the chemotherapy had worked well on me because my cancer is Triple-negative, not hormone related. My chemo is called 'Neoadjuvant' chemo, sometimes called 'primary medical treatment' and just means having the chemo *before* surgery. 'Adjuvant' alone means having it afterwards. To my mind it makes perfect sense to give patients who might respond well to chemo the treatment before surgery and thus shrink the tumour, making it smaller and easier to remove. Certainly with breasts it makes sense as, the smaller the dent in your boob, the better it will match with the other one. I know some poor patients decide to have cosmetic surgery after cancer surgery to make the healthy breast the same size as the operated one. Why has no one yet invented a bra with different sized cups each side? So many women, like me, have different sized right and left breasts even without cancer surgery making them even more different from each other. Different sized right and left cups would be more comfortable and would not particularly show under clothes. A job for Rigby and Peller, the Queen's corsetieres, perhaps?

ADVICE: Patricia warned that, as Triple-negative patients do not respond to and therefore cannot be treated with the usual drugs like Tamoxifen, they have to be extra careful that cancer does not return. She suggested having a blood test to measure my immune system six months after radiotherapy. Apparently you cannot get this on the NHS but personally I would be happy to pay to have the test regularly, just to be sure.

Patricia said to keep up the good work with the Cancer Diet and to have 'treats' but that 'moderation' is the key, rather than cutting out all your favourite foods forever – hooray! She felt I would sail through the lumpectomy but may be a bit sore from the sentinel node biopsy. She also mentioned that three to four weeks after surgery you can feel a few twinges when the cut nerves start to repair. She said I would have to wear a sports bra and lay off the tennis and bike riding for about a month after surgery but, hey, it will be jolly cold next month, so who cares!

WEDNESDAY 21ST NOVEMBER:
An Uplifting Message And Michelle Heaton

A routine consultation at the hospital today. Dr Hilary Martin could not find anything in my bust to measure – yay! She said they would organise a really experienced nurse to cannulate me tomorrow. Elena gave me a kiss and wished me well for my last chemo. Later that day there was a torrential downpour and afterwards the sky looked extraordinary. It was not just sky blue pink but vivid turquoise with banks of Turner-esque clouds and streaks of fuchsia. Sometimes this earth is so beautiful, it makes you think you so do not want to check out too soon!

When I got home I received a lovely email from a gentleman friend who had been in Australia and just discovered my situation. He wrote: *'I have to tell you, young lady, that with balloons up front or two fried eggs up front, NOTHING would detract from your beauty, your vibrance, your personality and your love of life. It's just THERE, it's not about any one part of you, it's about the whole and there is a helluva lot more to YOU that people love.'*

I was so touched that I shed a little tear. This is exactly what my lawyer pal Mike Cooper had said, that guys look at the whole package, not just one part of us. This is easy for me to say because I am now just having a lumpectomy but it is particularly valid for mastectomy patients.

Much has been written in the Press recently about the singer Michelle Heaton, who is apparently genetically 50–80% likely to get breast cancer and has just had a double mastectomy to prevent it, now while she is still young and fit. She has said it was very painful of course but she is glad to have done it. This is the 'prevention rather than cure' route and many people have been surprised at her decision, but one must respect her bravery. I wish her well.

THURSDAY 22ND NOVEMBER:
Last Chemo – yay!

Senior nurse Sally was supervising today, not treating, but found me a very experienced nurse called Valerie who gave me my Lorazepam and plunged my left arm into very hot water, then cannulated me quickly and easily in the same left front vein that had been so resistant last time.

ADVICE: *The anaesthetic gel I had been having to dull pain is cold and actually shrinks the veins, making them harder to cannulate. The hot water works just as well as an anaesthetic and opens up the veins. If you are having problems with your veins, it is worth waiting as long as it takes for an extremely experienced nurse. It is quicker for the hospital if the nurse gets the cannula in first time. The junior nurses need to practise but they can work on patients with better, fresher, newer veins. Somebody told me, 'A good chemo nurse can cannulate a brick!'*

Once cannulated, another nice nurse called Alice gave me my pre-meds very slowly (no prickly hedgehogs today!) and then the Taxol. Some mild discomfort in the vein was eased by a warm pad wrapped around the arm and I actually fell asleep for a good hour. Then it was over – I had finished my chemo course! I could not believe it and jumped up and down like Rylan (a very enthusiastic X-Factor contestant), kissing all the nurses and hugging Jade, my faithful chemo buddy. I am so happy, the time has gone by so fast.

SATURDAY 24TH NOVEMBER:
'The Anglistanis' And Larry Hagman

I was feeling OK this time, just my regular vein ache, which I guess will take a while to heal and cause a bit of insomnia and irritability. So I accepted a little filming job from my friend Eva Gray, playing an irate landlady in an independent film called *The Anglistanis*. There was only one scene with just a few lines and the acting part of it was easy. The keeping warm filming on a doorstep in pouring rain was more challenging and I raced home afterwards and jumped in a hot bath – no way am I getting another cold now I am leaving chemo behind me.

While watching TV in a café on location, director Ike Khan and I were sad to see that the legendary actor, Larry 'JR' Hagman had died aged 81 from complications following throat cancer. He was one of the most famous TV actors in the world and will be much missed. I feel a kinship with fellow cancer patients; I know how much Larry Hagman must have suffered with the treatments and the stress and I so admire him for carrying on working whilst still ill (the new *Dallas* has just finished airing on British TV). He was a true star right up until the very end. Goodbye, 'JR'.

TUESDAY 27TH NOVEMBER:
Brows And Lashes

I have now had my last three boosters from the district nurse. My health is all right, I am just a bit queasy and have had one small nosebleed but am looking forward to getting rid of the chemo side-effects permanently. My looks, how-ever, have taken a beating and today I dealt with my poor balding eyebrows and lashes. I toddled off to my beauty therapist, Kamini, and got my brows dyed, which immedi-ately made them look twice as thick.

ADVICE: *Kami advised me not to use regrowth potions on my brows, as those products can make them wiry. She suggested instead applying castor oil – well I never!*

My next stop was a local lash extension salon, Perfect Eyelashes, in London's Olympia, where they care for your lashes while they are growing back. The owner, Agnes, did my lashes herself, applying tiny little short ones which my own sparse lashes are able to support to give a natural look. She said wearing my usual long extensions or false lashes which I wear for my theatre work would damage the growing lashes and are a no-no for the moment but that, as my natural lashes regrow, she can give me longer ones if needed for work. As I am not working much at the moment, having cancelled my panto, I can concentrate on nurturing my baby lashes and hope that soon I will not need the extensions any more. For the moment my lashes look just like natural short ones – definitely a great improvement on practically bald! Agnes was very gentle and advised me to use RevitaLash lotion twice a day (safe with the extensions) and the RevitaLash mascara if I needed mascara on the bottom lashes. I had heard of RevitaLash: an American doctor, Dr Michael Brinkenhoff, had invented the product with some scientists when his wife Gayle had been deva-stated to lose her lashes during chemo. Happily her lashes had made a full recovery with the product. This is such a heart warming and indeed romantic story and inspired me to get some myself – fingers crossed!

THURSDAY 29TH NOVEMBER:
Celebrating And Fund-raising

Tonight I had a little party – in conjunction with *OK! Magazine*, of course! – to celebrate the end of my chemo course and raise funds for the cancer charity Yes to Life. Charlotte organised the party at the Millennium Mayfair Avista Bar (our second home!), Cetuem and Avista sponsored the function, and many of my friends and family turned up to wish me well. It was great to finally meet Robin and his colleague Sue from Yes to Life, and Patricia and Hayley from Cancer Options. Various of my cancer sufferer and cancer carer friends attended and there was a very warm and supportive atmosphere. Long-time friend Mark Field, the MP for Westminster, popped in to add the seal of approval with his wife Vicki and, with the help of Ingrid Tarrant in the raffle and Anna Brocklebank in the auction, we managed to raise a few grand for the charity. Even boxer Chris Eubank stuck his nose in to say 'hi' and give everyone a thrill.

FRIDAY 30th NOVEMBER:
The Disappearing Shrinking Tumours!

Today I had my end of chemo ultrasound with lady doctor, Dr Pope and my actual tumours, not counting the surrounding DCIS, appear to have shrunk to about 0.4 x 0.6 cm.

They will measure the exact amount when they open me up but it is looking really good – chemo truly works for my type of cancer. I was so happy with the news, I was walking on air; I am so blessed. Hopefully the operation will be routine with no nasties in the lymph, the radiotherapy will go well and I will be given the all clear in the spring. My feeling is very positive and I am euphoric.

SUNDAY 2ND DECEMBER:
Friends' Cancers And A Ray Of Hope

Today a sad truth hit home to me – not all cancer sufferers are as lucky as me and are able to have 'the killing treatment' (chemo). This morning I spoke to an old friend of mine in his early sixties who has sadly had a recurrence of cancer of the sacrum (the bony bit in the pelvic area). He was unable to have surgery or chemo for that area and has had as much radiotherapy as he can take, so has been put on a cocktail of pills. The poor chap is already limping and says that the cancer affects all the nerves in the area and he could end up in a wheelchair, incontinent, impotent and with a colostomy bag.

Then I checked in with another old friend, 'Pat From the Isle of Wight', who had survived breast cancer and a lumpectomy a few years ago. She had worn her lumpectomy scar with pride in evening dresses and we all thought she was cured. However, the cancer came back last year in her lungs and she had developed hypocalcemia, a condition which rots the calcium in your body: it had given her horribly itchy skin and she had dropped several stone in weight. Although, like my other friend, Pat is only in her early sixties, she has been told nothing can be done and has been given just months to live. She said the medics told her son David and he chose to tell her but that she is pleased to know the truth. This is ghastly and I immediately put both my friends in touch with Patricia at Cancer Options, 'bionic' Billy Carter and Christine, regarding the clinic in Dallas.

My friends' recent updates were very distressing but later that day there was a big ray of hope. I read a very interesting article by Lord Saatchi, who sadly lost his wife Josephine to peritoneal cancer, a rare form of the disease, in 2011. He wrote that he will be introducing the Medical Innovation Bill 2012 in the House of Lords tomorrow to change the way we treat patients, many of them terminally ill, in this country and ultimately to find a cure for cancer. He cannot believe that there is not yet a cure and believes innovative doctors have been put off by the fear of being sued for medical negligence. This new bill will protect doctors who want to try new and different treatments.

Lord Saatchi makes the point that the current treatments available – invasive surgery, chemo and radio – do not always work and that chemo particularly creates the same symptoms as the disease and damages the immune system, which can open a path to fatal infection. I am just one little person who knows these facts from experience and I will be rooting for this Bill to go through. Let us hope that because of this Bill many cancer patients, including my own friends who are classed as terminal or have been told nothing more can be done for them, will now have reprieves.

For myself, I just have a cold and the usual insomnia, which makes me very irritable (I completely lost it with the surly so-and-so on my Tesco Local checkout, who dropped not one, but two of my soups yesterday – splat!).

I had a drink with my very fit pal Prince Alexander

Bassey – who has a friend who's also struggling through breast cancer and chemo – and his personal trainer Ruthy – who is a fitness and nutritional expert – and we discussed the cocktail of supplements Patricia has designed for me. Ruthy reckons they will work well and said that the magnesium particularly should help my insomnia – jolly good because I would not want to be 'persona non grata' in all the local supermarkets! Ruthy also said that coffee was OK, which is a relief because, although I am drinking it because it is 'good' for cancer, I am not really mad about the famous green tea.

WEDNESDAY 5TH DECEMBER:
Preparing For Surgery

Today was a day of running around the hospital, taking my clothes off and putting them back on again! First I saw the reassuring Mr Gui, who was very pleased with the shrinkage of the tumours and said it was full steam ahead for the wide local excision and sentinel node biopsy on the 13th. He gave me a choice of scar positions and I chose to have two small scars, one on the aureole and one under the arm, rather than one longer one down the side of the breast – always provided that was possible when he opened me up.

Interestingly, Mr Gui said that Professor Smith might try me on Tamoxifen after radiotherapy as, although I had always been described as 'Triple-negative' after my original core biopsy, my oestrogen level then was actually three out of eight, whereas my progesterone and HER2 were nought out of eight. I have no idea what it all means but am

179

prepared to try anything. I understand that I responded well to chemo because my cancer was *not* hormonally driven, but that Tamoxifen only works on 'positive' patients. However three out of eight is almost half, so who knows? At the moment I must just concentrate on getting through the surgery.

Next I went off to another part of the hospital to have my bazookas photographed – they snap them both in case you need any 'even-ing up' of the healthy breast after the diseased one has been operated on. Mine are pretty asymmetric anyway! The kindly photographer was handicapped (maybe a former Thalidomide patient?), God bless him, and seeing him wield the camera so dexterously with tiny arms was inspiring and humbling. But I didn't have time to think about him for long as I had to race off to Surgical Admissions on the first floor where staff nurse Eleanor and nurse Erika looked after me. They sent me off for a blood test and did the usual swabbing, blood pressure, height and weight, etc. Then – new tricks – they gave me an ECG, where they put lots of pads all over my body to check that my heart was up to surgery. My heart is – my emotions, not so much! I am nervous and apprehensive and just want to get the surgery over with – still, only eight days to go now.

SATURDAY 8TH DECEMBER:
Lymph Glands, Billy And Neon

I met a glamorous Middle Eastern lady at a party who told me that she too had had surgery, chemo and radio for breast cancer.

ADVICE: This lady advised not to have all my lymph glands removed 'just in case', if they were non-cancerous. She said that she had requested to have all of hers removed along with her lumpectomy for safety but that she had then had lymphodoema (swelling) and lymphatic drainage problems. Two years later she was still swollen, especially in her ankles, and believed it was lymphatic drainage problems – although she was still on Tamoxifen, which can make you put on weight.

On the plus side she looked great with long, lustrous hair which she said had grown back to its original length in just two years (however, dark, Middle Eastern hair is stronger than European hair). Her nastiest chemo side-effects – acidity and haemorrhoids – had disappeared in a matter of months and her lashes and brows had gradually grown back. Her veins had gone dark and swollen like mine but had recovered after eight months. Happily this lady now seemed fit and healthy and said her actual lumpectomy operation had been fine, which calmed me down a bit!

ADVICE: She had managed to cover her 'chemo veins' with foundation and lots of bangles.

I received a huge Christmas card from 'Bionic Billy' Carter, with a round robin, agonised plea for doctors to find a cure for cancer so that patients could live safely with the disease. He made the valid point that that is what had happened for AIDS/HIV patients when the disease had first become rife in the Eighties. Those AIDS/HIV patients can now live comfortably with medication thanks to medical genius, whereas we are losing cancer patients all the time.

In the news at the moment is the heart-rending case of mum Sally Roberts, who kidnapped her seven-year-old son Neon to prevent him being given radiotherapy after brain tumour surgery. She had panicked after an insensitive doctor had talked about 'frying Neon's brain' with radio-therapy and she had actually gone to court over it as she said she feared the treatment could affect Neon's IQ and make him infertile, amongst other things. Sadly the cancer had returned and the poor young lad had to have more surgery with the possibility of both chemo and radiotherapy in the future. It is an absolute tragedy when cancer hits kids so young.

WEDNESDAY 12TH DECEMBER:
Sentinel Node Injection And Scan

In fear and trembling I tottered off to the main radiology department on the fourth floor of the Marsden, where a technician called Catherine looked after me. I had been very nervous about the injection for the scan as it had to be put into the sensitive aureole, and it was impossible to have any numbing cream for it. However, it really was not too bad. Catherine was very gentle and it just felt like a bee sting for a few seconds – at least what I imagine a bee sting to feel like, as I have never been stung!

The injection puts a fluid, presumably with a dye, into the lymph to show the lymphatic drainage of the breast and give the surgeon a 'map' of where to find the lymph nodes to test during surgery. After the injection Catherine mas-saged the injected area gently to spread the fluid, then proceeded with three, five-minute scans where everything showed up fine. My lymph node 'map' was now in position. I am terrified at the thought that some of my lymph nodes might also be cancerous but at least I will know soon.

Today I also met Matthew, a helpful young trainee surgeon on Mr Gui's team. I had had one of my usual swollen glands/head colds and had been taking Amoxicillin once again, so I was worried that I might not be fit for surgery. However Matthew listened to my chest and back and pronounced me fine – so there was no getting out of it!

THURSDAY 13TH DECEMBER: *Surgery Day!*

Jade was working this morning but Jeremy dropped me at the Marsden at 7.45am and I went up to the Day Surgery Unit. Mr Gui and his surgical team all came to see me, plus the lady anaesthetist. At 9.15am I had an ultrasound to mark up the area to be excised. The kind imaging doctor asked me how I felt and I said, 'Very nervous'. He said, 'Don't worry, you are in the best hands'. I know I am with Mr Gui, because his reputation has preceeded him, but I am still nervous about the anaesthetic.

I had kept myself busy during the last week, going down to Longleat in Wiltshire for lunch, seeing lots of friends and attending a round of BAFTA films, so I was nicely tired, which took the edge off my panic.

ADVICE: *Take a book or something to do if you are by yourself to take your mind off your impending surgery. There is always waiting-around time. The anaesthetist and surgeon are duty bound to warn you of all the things that could go wrong – waking up during the operation, having to have more surgery if they find more cancer, etc – and of course it is scary but just KEEP CALM!*

I've never had an operation on the NHS before. I'd gone privately when having Jade, my appendectomy and my eyes implanted (a very clever op I had had at Optical Express in Westfields earlier in the year when they replaced the lenses inside my astigmatic eyes with brand new better than 20/20 vision ones!), but it was brilliant, they all looked after me so well. Staff nurse Eleanor and nurse Erika kitted me out with frilly, disposable knicks, anti-swelling socks and slipper-socks, then it was into my gown and robe and down to theatre at around 11.30.

I'd always wondered why it was called 'theatre' and theatre nurse Sandy explained that in the old days surgeons, who had originally been barbers, performed their operations in a big space like a Greek amphitheatre, with spectators looking on interestedly at the blood and gore! Luckily my theatre today was small and neat. Mr Gui came in to tell me it was unlikely that my sentinel lymph node biopsy would be positive (he had obviously noticed me going rigid with fear, bless him!). Then the lady anaesthetist, Dr Fiona McManus, arrived and I gulped. In fact the anaesthesia was sheer perfection. I had had some anaesthetic gel put onto the injection site earlier and all I felt was a tiny scratch in my wrist. One moment Fiona and I were chatting about the colour of our eyes and the length of Sandy's eyelashes and the next I was waking up, all done!

I had a small amount of pain in my boob, which was instantly fixed through the drip and then I was stretchered back up to the Day Surgery Unit. Someone then told me my sentinel lymph node biopsy had been negative – YESSSSS!

I was thrilled to find Jade upstairs waiting for me with a bunch of gorgeous fresh roses; she had located me by spotting my shoes in my cubicle and the nurses had realised she was my daughter from our resemblance. It was an ecstatic reunion. Surgeon Ana Agusti and some of the Gui surgical team came round and told me that all was well, the tumours had been excised, the scars were where I had requested them and the sentinel node had indeed been negative. She said Mr Gui, who was by then operating on another patient, had looked at a couple of other nodes but I was too woozy for them to go into it in more depth.

After being checked and having something to eat and drink, I was free to go. I had smallish dressings on the breast and underarm and put a sports bra over them. My brother, Crock, had come to collect us and it was off home to recuperate.

I have to give the Marsden 10 out of 10 for my operation; the hospital so deserves its brilliant reputation. The nursing care, the anaesthesia and, of course, the surgery, were all exemplary. I feel truly blessed and so lucky that it seems the cancer has definitely not spread.

SATURDAY 15TH DECEMBER:
Comfort And Sadness

My wounds were pretty comfortable and I have not needed the painkillers I was sent home with. Kate Jones, the

Marsden physio, had sent me some exercises to do to regain or maintain full use of my arm and shoulder quickly after the operation on the axilla (armpit) and I was managing them fairly well. On Patricia Peat's advice I was trying a Melatonin under-tongue spray for my ongoing insomnia and cold remedies for my ongoing cold and cough and keeping warm indoors.

Then I received some terrible news. Micee, a girlfriend I had met through Pat Duncan and bumped into at tennis occasionally, had died after falling down the stairs at home and cutting her head. She was not old and quite fit, so it was a dreadful shock to her poor young son and husband, whom I spoke to on the phone. A tragedy. We fight so hard for our little lives but they can be snuffed out in an instant, seemingly without rhyme or reason.

FRIDAY 21ST DECEMBER:
Post-Op Check-up

After a comfortable week not having to take a single painkiller, I returned to Mr Gui's clinic in General Outpatients. In Mr Gui's absence I saw a lady doctor, who had very good news for me: all the cancer had been excised, the other two lymph nodes Mr Gui had looked at were negative (apparently they usually are if the sentinel node is negative) and there was no seroma (fluid) leaking from the lymph. HOORAY! I am so happy, this is the best ever Christmas present for my family and myself. I am so blessed.

Then I had a long chat with nurse Vanda, who took my dressings off, leaving me with just small Steri-strips on the actual wounds, which she said would come off of their own accord with bathing, etc. Vanda said I could go back to driving after two to three weeks and do my regular stomach and leg exercises immediately, as long as I left out the arm ones and stuck to my physio exercises. Now the dressings were off, I could immediately move my arms around more comfortably and look forward to returning to my tennis and cycling, although Vanda did say I might have to miss skiing this year – a small price to pay for excising the cancer successfully.

For the future, Vanda said I would see the radiologists in a few weeks' time and start my radiotherapy course after consultation with them. She said she was not sure whether I would go on Tamoxifen afterwards or not. The tumours had been tested again after their removal and they would see if the results were the same as the original biopsy, i.e. three out of eight oestrogen, and both progesterone and HER2 completely negative. If I did not go on the pills I would just have to be vigilant to make sure the cancer did not return. I would have a mammogram once a year but, remembering that my little speck in 2011 had turned into 3 centimetres of cancerous tumours a year later, I am determined to protect myself from breast and all cancer with the Cancer Diet, general lifestyle, less stress and the six-monthly immune system check-ups that Patricia Peat of Cancer Options suggested.

Whatever the future holds, I am clear at the moment and I wafted round the hospital in a state of euphoria, chatting to Geraldine and Elena who were both thrilled for me, God bless their kind hearts.

I decided it was celebration time and my favourite escort

(and I mean that in the nicest possible way!) Mike Cooper and I trotted off to a couple of parties, firstly for drinks hosted by Lalla Kaur and Michael Gelardi at The Mayfair Hotel to celebrate Michael's birthday, and then to Louise Hyam's beautiful flat in Regent's Park for a supper party for my old mate Donald Stewart, who was visiting from Italy.

Donald's three grown-up daughters – Georgina, Jessica and Antonia – were there and Georgina told me that their mum had sadly died of breast cancer ten years ago at the age of sixty-two, after fighting it for eight years. She said that her mum had undergone all sorts of research tests which she believed helped breast cancer patients of today, such as me, to survive. This made me terribly sad and I burst into tears. Georgina hugged me and said it was OK and that she was so happy for me. A brave and generous girl. I just hope that Dr Turner's research involving regular blood tests and the Chemonia Research Yukie and her colleagues have done on me (seeing how chemo affects the tumours by giving patients regular tests) will also help future patients and save more lives.

The scientists and medics are learning more about cancer all the time. A lady whose best friend happily survived breast cancer recently kindly sent me the following interesting news about how you can easily protect yourself from thyroid cancer:

'On Wednesday, Dr. Oz had a show on the fastest growing cancer in women, thyroid cancer. It was a very interesting programme and he mentioned that the increase could possibly be related to the use of dental X-rays and mammograms. He demonstrated that on the apron the dentist puts on you for *your dental X-rays there is a little flap that can be lifted up and wrapped around your neck. Many dentists don't bother to use it. Also, there is something called a "thyroid guard" for use during mammograms. By coincidence, I had my yearly mammogram yesterday. I felt a little silly, but I asked about the guard and sure enough, the technician had one in a drawer. I asked why it wasn't routinely used. Answer: "I don't know. You have to ask for it." Well, if I hadn't seen the show, how would I have known to ask? We need to pass this on to our daughters, nieces, mothers and all our female friends and, husbands, tell your wives!'*

I had not heard of Dr Oz before and when I asked my very efficient dentist Mr Malcolm Freiberger about this he said the negligible amount of radiation you get from dental X-rays could never cause cancer. Maybe this is true with mammograms too. However it cannot hurt to protect oneself and, if it makes you feel safer, why not do it?

I have never really approved of animal testing but, if it can save human lives, I have to accept it. Having lost three male friends, including our much loved 'Nanny Geoff' to prostate cancer, I thought the following very valuable:

From: NHS Choices
Sent: Friday, December 21, 2012 7:27am
Subject: 'Trojan horse' cancer therapy could be effective.
BBC News reports that an experimental therapy hides 'cancer killing viruses inside the immune system in order to sneak them into a tumour' and that this Trojan-horse therapy 'completely eliminates' cancer in mice.
This news is based on early-stage research into a new type of

cancer treatment, using viruses to target and attack cancerous tumours. Several research teams have adopted this approach in recent years. The current study took advantage of large immune system cells called macrophages that increase in number in the tumour after standard chemotherapy and radiation treatment.

The scientists treated mice that had prostate cancer with chemotherapy, and then used these immune system cells to deliver a virus to the remaining tumour. This virus then multiplied and attacked the tumour cells. Compared to mice who received the chemotherapy only, those who received the additional treatment lived longer and did not experience any spreading of the tumour beyond the prostate.

This research provides early evidence that using the immune system's existing cells may offer a mechanism by which to deliver novel cancer treatments. This research is still in its early stages, and trials in people will be needed to ensure that the approach is safe and effective for treating human prostate cancer.'

Well, I just hope they get on with it!

THURSDAY 27TH DECEMBER:
Getting On With It – Hair And Make-up

Christmas was very happy for us all and I was very spoiled, going to family and friends and being cooked for.

ADVICE: Health-wise, everything is hunky-dory and I am working on my immune system with supplements and my *insomnia with Melatonin spray but looks-wise I can tell it will be a while (and I have to wonder if ever) before I get back to normal. My hair never went completely bald but patchy bald, so Steven shaved it for me to help it grow back uniformly. However, my scalp then felt more itchy with the wig on, so he then had to get me some spirit gum and remover from Angel's theatrical costumiers for the next stage of wiggery: using the wig cap. I already had wig caps from my theatrical work and was able to glue the wig to the wig cap securely and comfortably, removing the gum with the remover.*

On Boxing Day at my friend Dr Anna's, I sat next to her brother Billy, a top surgeon who said, 'You can tell the NHS wigs a mile off!' Anna and I giggled and introduced him to Crystal. He was absolutely shocked and gobsmacked and had to feel the wig, as had Professor Smith when I first unveiled Crystal. It does not feel as silky as just-washed real hair but Anna made the point that acrylic wigs actually feel no different from real hair with hairspray and other products on.

My brows are still very sparse and I have no lashes whatsoever on my upper right eye (weird – we had a teacher at school with no lashes and we laughed at her, horrid little girls that we were – now I've had my come-uppance!) and about three on my left, with about three on each lower eyelid. So there are no lashes to attach the individual lashes on to and I have to wear strip lashes, attached to the skin of the eyelid, all the time now if I want to continue to look like me!

Harriet, a pretty young girl working on the Dior counter in Harrods, admired my make-up while I was Christmas shopping last week and I was thrilled that someone actually in the make-up business could appreciate my 'bald face' disguise! Chemo patients with no hair, lashes and brows should not have to cover themselves up if they do not want to. There is no shame and much bravery in going through chemo and others should respect that. But if you do want to disguise your chemo look (or maybe *have* to for your job), here are the products I used:

* Natural Image acrylic wig 'Crystal'

* Nails Inc Strip Lashes (but you can get all sorts of good lashes just about everywhere nowadays)

* Revitalash mascara, to revive what little you have left whilst still colouring and lengthening

* L'Oreal powder eyeshadow for above and below eyes and for the brows and L'Oreal eye and lip lining pencils (all kindly given to me by the charity Look Good... Feel Better).

*BeauBronz Abi O Soft Sun Self Tan and Skin Perfekt Skin Perfection Gel in Radiant, to subtly cover your pallor

* Estée Lauder Pure Colour Blush (this is expensive but Jade sweetly got it for me – 'phone a friend'!)

* My lips have been very dry ever since I started chemo so, unless I have to wear lippy for something special, I tend to use lip salve with a bit of lip pencil round the outside for definition.

WEDNESDAY 2ND JANUARY 2013: *Happy New Year!*

Thank God last year's over, truly an Annus Horribilis for *moi*. I had a quiet New Year's Eve with family and friends and resolved to be healthier and tougher this year. I am feeling OK – no cold for several days, which is a result! Jeremy is kindly funding my drug supplements habit at The Nutri Centre and I am taking the biggest, strongest vitamins and minerals I can find.

ADVICE: *if you find it hard to swallow your supplements, try taking them with food rather than water – or cut them into smaller bits.*

To maintain the mobility in my arm and shoulder I am doing my physio exercises. The first two sets were a doddle but I overdid the third lot, which involved stretching, and made my arm and shoulder hurt (the rotator cuff?) – idiot! I spoke to Kate, the Marsden physio, and she advised me to return to the second, easier exercises until my arm and shoulder were feeling more comfortable.

ADVICE: *take it easy with the physio stretches – you just need mobility, not longer arms!*

Looks-wise, my scars are small but not pleasant and there is a big pad of fat hanging over the dent where the lymph gland was removed. Watching the *Sex And The City* 1 film (as one does at New Year) I decided I may have to opt for the Vivienne Westwood 'Carrie' wedding dress look, which has crafty pointed bits under the armpits. But hey, I am not one to complain and am delighted to be cancer free and regaining my strength. An old friend who only rings once a year to wish me many happies said he had had a 'boys' problem' last year but was getting over it. I was delighted to be able to reply that I had had a 'girls' problem' but was also getting over it. Because I am.

Jadey is staying with her best friend Minnie Kemp and her family in Barbados, hobnobbing with the likes of Simon Cowell AND Andrew Lloyd Webber (I do love a good name-drop!) so I borrowed her huge and gorgeous furry cap to give Crystal a rest, put eye shadow round my lashless eyes and toddled off, in the car at last, to get my break-y, flakey nails done at Harvey Nichs, which cheered me up no end. The long-lashed Lauren (I am so jealous) said my nails were starting to grow back and I could now have porous gel varnish instead of the covering gel business. This is a minor but happy little triumph for me. First the nails, next the hair and lashes – and, oh yes, the brows!

THURSDAY 3RD JANUARY:
Death And Life

Today was the funeral of Micee, the poor lady who had fallen down the stairs and tragically died after cracking her head open. The service was at Holy Trinity Brompton and her devoted son Robert gave his mum a wonderful tribute. The priest told us that 'death is inevitable' and we all know that but it is still so hard for those who are left behind.

I drove home feeling sad, then received a cheerful email from Fabia, a fun burlesque artiste famous for her light-up tassels on *Britain's Got Talent*. Fabia supports a breast cancer charity and we had been emailing each other after meeting through Steve and Diane, the lovely couple behind one of my favourite endorsements, *Bags Of Dreams*. She said she had read my latest Hot Gossip column where I had included a snap of my palm and invited 'readings', and said: 'Your palm shows a long life line'. Thanks, Fabia, I am working on it!

MONDAY 7TH JANUARY:
Seeing Linda

I went for my first casting from my new agent, Rob Groves (my previous long-time agent, Michele Hart, having just retired). It was for a Comic Relief commercial and, although I never heard a word (obviously I do not look enough like the iconic Farrah Fawcett for this part!), I was thrilled to bump into my old mate Linda Regan and have a coffee and a catch-up. Linda and I first worked together in 1980 in Tom Stoppard's hilarious *Dirty Linen* and once got locked in the – allegedly haunted – Arts Theatre in the dark until rescued by the police – ah, happy days!

Linda, a very kind lady, advised me that she had various actress pals who had sadly had cancer and lost work when producers had not been able to insure them. I will just have to hope that, after radiotherapy, I will get the all-clear and be insurable again. At the moment Rob can only look for small jobs for me. Poor Linda had lost good friends to 'the big C' like me and we had some sad moments remembering them all.

WEDNESDAY 9TH JANUARY:
Scars And Insomnia

ADVICE: I had a phone consultation with Patricia Peat from Cancer Options about my scars. The scars are good, small ones (thank you, Mr Gui): the one on my bust does not show but the lymph gland one is above the level of many of my evening dresses and I needed to know when I could start applying anti-scarring potions. My close and caring friends Patrick and Annabel Curtis had kindly sent me some Scar-guard, which has Vitamin E in it, from the States, and Patricia said that that product or any with Vitamin E would be good and I could start applying it now, twenty-eight days after surgery.

That night I enjoyed a fun 'Supper with Sally' charity dinner at Avista, with Charlotte and Paddy and Sheena Evershed, hosted and organised by dynamic duo Anna Brocklebank and Ingrid Tarrant, and kind Ingrid promised to find me an aloe vera plant. The fresh juice of the plant is amazingly healing and brilliant for scars.

ADVICE: Patricia had also advised me to use my melatonin spray (to counteract my insomnia) every night for two weeks to encourage my body to produce its own melatonin and tonight I started my fortnight's course. I had only used it occasionally, silly me – always read the instructions!

THURSDAY 10TH JANUARY:
Lashes And Things

ADVICE: EYELASH REGROWTH. This morning – seven weeks after the end of my chemo course – I was totally thrilled when I peered in the mirror and noticed little stubby baby lashes sprouting on my lower eyelids! My lashes had *completely disappeared, top and bottom, but I had started using Rapid Lash from Boots, as advised by Jill at The Haven LGFB (Look Good...Feel Better) seminar, on my bottom ones. (At £41, it is expensive and I can hide my upper lash baldness with strip lashes, so I had just used it on the bottom – lo and behold, the bottom lashes had grown and not the top ones.) The little lashes are adorable and I could not stop stroking them!*

My hair has also sprouted a bit on top, maybe thanks to my nightly application of Cetuem treatment spray, but is still very bald at the sides and back.

Later that day I ran in to one of my neighbours, an attractive lady who had just turned fifty. She said that she had been diagnosed with the horrid ovarian cancer last year, had a seven-hour operation and then a course of chemo, also at the Marsden. She was still on Taxol but not having many side-effects, just a bit of tingling, like I had had. Her hair was still thick and lustrous. I wonder which cancer chemo treatments you lose your hair with and which you do not? Certainly you almost always do with breast cancer chemo.

A strong lady, she was getting through it and her cancer marker had gone down considerably. However she said her daughter, aged twenty-one like Jade, had not been strong enough to attend chemo, surgery and consultations with her. Poor thing, I do understand – you see such sad cases at the hospital, it must be so hard for the 'carers'. I felt so blessed that my Jadey had been so strong for me, and I offered to accompany my neighbour to her chemo sessions in future if she did not find anyone better.

That evening my healer, David Goodman, came over for a session. He worked on my general health and recovery after excising the cancer tumours, my – sore from overdoing the physio exercises – arm and shoulder and the swift healing of my scars. I felt brilliant afterwards and slept really well too; David is excellent. I am so lucky to have my little team around me: David, Patricia Peat from Cancer Options, Lucien my hypno and Peter Cox, my nutritionist.

I also had a lovely message from Mark Moody today after I had thanked him for regularly including my picture in his *Ok!* column and saying I did not want people to forget me because I was ill. Mark replied, 'No one could ever forget you, Sally'. Bless him, it's the little kindnesses that make you cry.

TUESDAY 15TH JANUARY:
Springtime In Lashland

Eureka! Today, approximately seven-and-a-half weeks after finishing chemo, I noticed that my upper eyelids are also sprouting little baby lashes – and my eyebrows are growing back really fast. This is all wonderful but the downside is that my moustache is also reappearing! Oh well, at least Kamini the Eyebrow Queen will be welcoming me back for the threading business – I wonder if she has missed me?

THURSDAY 17TH JANUARY:
Spiritual Healing

After the success of Lucien's hypnotherapy with my needle and blood phobias, he had now started working on my insomnia to complement the melatonin spray. Lucien had suggested that I try some spiritual healing for my psyche. Well, I am game for anything these days so trotted off to meet him and his pal Lucia at The Spiritualist Association of Great Britain in Victoria. I am not into mediums after a useless experience with one but healing is healing and if the practitioner is good, I am sure it helps. In the event a lady called Anne gave me the healing and I know it helped me. All the healers wore white coats and you did not have to pay, just donate whatever amount you wanted into a collection box, which I thought was very ethical. I did not feel anything at first but about half an hour after the twenty-minute session I started to feel very happy. I slept really well that night too.

SUNDAY 20TH JANUARY:
Being Pro-active – Diana's Story

Today I had a long chat with Diana, a very brave cancer survivor and Yes To Life helpline volunteer. Poor Diana had really been through a traumatic time with her cancer treatment.

Six years ago, when she was 47, she had found a lump which for over six months her local hospital thought was a cyst. They had been unable to drain it and Diana had caught an agonising infection and swelling from the needle. A biopsy had proved ambiguous but they decided they should remove the lump anyway. This was done at the local hospital, after which Grade 2 cancer was confirmed, so they then wanted to remove all of Diana's lymph glands, which worried her a lot, as they said they didn't think the cancer had spread but said there was a 15-20% chance of this surgery causing lymphodema.

So she was referred to a top cancer hospital, where she could have a Sentinel Node Biopsy, so that just 4 lymph nodes were removed (which turned out to be non-cancerous as expected), instead of all of them. Sadly this was not the happy ending to the story. The hospital, with no explanation, decided that her tumour was Grade 3 not 2, and they wanted her to have chemotherapy as well.

She feels that the chemo had a devastating effect on her future health.

She was prescribed 12 half doses of FEC chemo, rather than 6 full ones, designed to minimise side-effects. However, this meant she had to endure more treatments, and had less recovery time in between. She had felt so sick that she had been unable to prepare food at all and her constipation resulting from Granisetron, an anti-sickness drug injected before each chemo, had been so bad that she had torn her rectum. She said that going to the loo felt like 'passing broken glass' and that this effect lasted for several months after the chemo was finished and she also became incontinent. The pain and suffering of this poor woman is humbling.

The 'shotty in the botty' single immune system boosting injection had given her terrible back pain so she had had to have lower dose shots on successive days. Interestingly, the one thing Diana <u>did</u> save was her long hair, although it got thinner.

ADVICE: HAIR LOSS AND THE ICE CAP: Diana believes what saved her hair was putting the ice cap on half an hour *extra before chemo, leaving it on for half an hour extra afterwards and having the cap changed not just once but twice. She lost every hair on her body, but not on her head. Good for her, she must have been frozen, but her bravery and determination saved her hair.*

However, after all her treatments were finished, Diana sadly did not get better. Her immune system was understandably shot by the chemo, she lost 2 stone in weight in 2 months (she was already very slim) and had continuous diarrhoea and breathing problems (she had always had mild asthma, but now was sometimes bedridden for days on end). She was coughing up blood, and at one stage her lung collapsed. She was severely allergic to any damp or mould, and had started to suffer from multiple chemical sensitivity, with normal household chemicals and toiletries triggering severe asthma attacks. She had candida and fungal and bacterial infections throughout her body, as a result of her low immunity following the chemo. These infections, she believes, were responsible for most of her other symptoms.

Hospital tests revealed no cancer, but the only thing the doctors had to offer for her multiple problems was more drugs, even though she was allergic to these! Diana was horrified at the lack of knowledge and support from her doctors, and she believes she would have died if she had not then become very pro-active and taken responsibility for her own health. She started to follow a strict organic wholefood diet, that was both anti-fungal and immune boosting, giving up all forms of sugar, wheat and gluten, dairy, all processed food, alcohol and started taking lots of natural supplements. She made her own fresh juices. All household chemicals and toiletries were removed from her home and replaced with natural alternatives.

She found Chris Woollen's Cancer Active and Patricia Peat's Cancer Options sites, Yes to Life, and studied cancer and natural health wherever she could and took advice from practitioners. She has since followed a naturapathic, holistic lifestyle, giving up unhealthy foods, taking no medical drugs whatsoever and having healing, acupuncture, shiatsu and other therapies. Most importantly, she has detoxified her body by a series of juice fasts, colon and liver cleanses, Far Infra Red saunas, skin brushing, Epsom salt baths, etc.

Diana's lifestyle changes brought immediate and dramatic improvements to her health. She has happily been clear of cancer for over 5 years now and has eliminated most of the horrific effects of the cancer treatment. She is getting healthier every day due to her excellent, disciplined lifestyle and was on good form when I met her with Robin Daly recently. She admits that she has never been a great exerciser and that this can have made a difference to her recovery. However, she really feels that she was pressurised into chemo by the docs and that the killing treatment caused all of her problems. She said that, if she had her time again, she would *never* have had the debilitating chemo and radiotherapies, just do everything natural to strengthen and rebuild her body so it could heal itself, rather than destroy it with devastating and toxic treatments.

A salutary story; an extraordinarily brave and inspirational lady who took charge of her life and cured herself of multiple health problems the natural way.

MONDAY 21ST JANUARY:
Radiotherapy Consultation

I saw friendly radiologists Dr Paolo De-Ieso and Dr Gillian Ross at the Marsden today. A hospital letter after surgery had confirmed that my original 2.5–3 centimetre tumours had shrunk with chemo to just 1 centimetre (1.5 including the area of pre-cancerous–only DCIS around the tumours). This is what they had found when they had opened me up and measured the areas exactly, being able to be more precise than the ultrasound scan. So the dreaded chemo had really done its stuff with the shrinkage.

I discussed this with Paolo and he explained that having radiotherapy after chemo and surgery would stop the breast cancer returning to 'My Left Boob' – hooray!

He said that if you have the whole breast removed by mastectomy there is no need for radiotherapy but that a lumpectomy and radiotherapy will have the same effect as a mastectomy, ie: prevent the cancer returning. I am so so so happy that I was able to have the much less invasive operation. The radiotherapy would take four weeks, Paolo said, going to the hospital every day in the weekdays, but it would only be for 15 minutes at a time and it would <u>not</u> hurt! So, remembering that I had not had to take a single painkiller after my surgery, I would so recommend having the lesser operation if you can. Thank you, Professor Smith for shrinking my tumours and Mr Gui for my painless surgery.

Paolo told me that I would have a CT scan this week to determine exactly where the lump was removed and then radio would start two weeks later. The radiologist would aim beams at the area from both sides; where the beams met in the middle was the cancer site. (The first three weeks I would have external treatment to the whole breast and the fourth week would be a 'booster' to the exact lump site.)

The doctors have to warn you that there are minimal risks of radiotherapy affecting your ribs (in the long run), lungs, heart (if the tumours were in the left breast, like mine) and of causing a second malignancy (a 1 in 10,000 chance). However, these things are extremely unlikely to happen. What _may_ happen is redness, tenderness and hardness and I would probably get quite tired, both during the month of treatment and for a month afterwards. But no real pain as such – yippee!

After my consultation, my brother and sister-in-law came to take me to lunch and were very impressed with this, their first view of the Marsden. 'It's spotlessly clean,' said Caroline. My injured breast puffed up with pride like a little bird – this was 'my' hospital, I had chosen it and it had proved to be such a good choice.

We went to lunch at a Thai restaurant called Patara near the hospital, where we had nice poached salmon, green tea and water from a glass bottle – all very healthy. Caroline said that Waitrose were now doing very good prepared mackerel – could be a change from the ubiquitous salmon! We discussed my new Brita water filter, which Patricia Peat had recommended and which Jeremy had been coerced into giving me for Christmas. Filtering tap water makes it safe to drink and it is obviously much cheaper than bottled water, you just have to replace the filter block every month.

ADVICE: *David and Caroline, who also have a water filter and swear by it, advised me to always pour away the old water*

when refilling the jug and to always wash all the parts of the
gadget scrupulously when replacing the filter.

That evening I met up with Ruth Sherratt and 'bionic'
Janie Martel and her friend 'Captain Kit' at Bar Boulud in
Knightsbridge. Ruth was on great form and it was wonderful
to finally meet Janie, who lives in Somerset, after many
phone calls and emails. Janie is not just a breast cancer
patient but also lives with brain damage and Addison's
(adrenal problems) but she is so bright and lively, no one
would ever know. I find her totally inspirational and it was
she who (along with many others) suggested Professor
Smith at the Marsden and Patricia Peat at Cancer Options
(the people who literally saved my life), not to mention
Robin Daly at Yes To Life, so I will always be eternally
grateful to her. Ruth was the darling who took me out and
cheered me up the day I was first diagnosed.

We had a lovely evening. Janie, like me, had been advised
to drink champagne and red wine, not white, so of course
we had to have plenty! Ruth and I ate chicken with lots of
fresh vegetables and Janie had salad whereas Captain Kit,
who is much older and probably much healthier than all of
us, tucked into red meat.

That night, in spite of sleeping better, I had one of my
regular anxiety dreams where I am looking for a school,
which is just around the corner. I know where it is but I can
never quite find it and run around like a headless chicken...
then it morphed into talking about scuba diving in the
South China Seas (do they scuba dive there?). All very weird
– as I said before, I can only conclude that I am anxious
now that I am so close to the finishing line and do not want

anything to go wrong. Lucien had advised me to recall my dreams for analysis. I do not usually remember them but that one was vivid.

THURSDAY 24TH JANUARY:
CT Scan

When I arrived at Radiology, the nice receptionist Jackie said. 'You look much more beautiful in the flesh than in photos'. I nearly burst into tears. I have been feeling quite down about my hair (it is growing back darker, greyer and wirier, as many people told me it would), and I now have stumpy lashes, pallor, scars, a 'dippy' boob and the extra 'expression lines' the stress of it all has given me. What a kind lady – and it means my wig and make-up are working well in covering up my imperfections!

ADVICE: *if you can give a cancer/chemo patient a genuine compliment, please do. From talking to other patients, I know that looks are important to us ladies and they sure are affected by chemo and surgery.*

The CT scan was fine. Radio superintendant Mandy and radiographer Craig looked after me very well. Mandy explained what would happen in detail and away we went. A CT scan does *not* hurt! There is a lot of fiddling about getting you into position with your arm up and the relevant bazooka sticking out, then covering your scars with wires and putting stickers on, then you go into a sort of short open tunnel – not at all claustrophobic – and lie still for five minutes, which is easy. It was a bit cold, though, and I had to concentrate on not sneezing so as not to move my body.

ADVICE: *To stop yourself sneezing, look down (if you do want to sneeze and get it over with, look up.)*

After the actual scan, Craig put permanent tattoos on three points of the breast so that the radiographer can position the beams exactly each time. This was not painful, just like little scratches from brambles, and the marks are very small and easily coverable with make-up. Apparently they do fade somewhat with time, according to other radio patients. Then I was given my radio dates, beginning 7th February for one month, and off I toddled.

I got lost coming out of the hospital and emerged in the MDU, scene of my chemo days. It was weird seeing all the equipment and remembering everything that had happened there – my hair, my veins, the last time I saw the amazing Ina on her feet. There is a nice male receptionist at MDU and I smiled at him – I guess he has seen a lot in that unit. Then I bumped into Geraldine, Professor Smith's lovely P.A., and was happy to report light at the end of my personal tunnel.

SUNDAY 27TH JANUARY:
Breast Cancer Research At A Ball!

Debbie Arnold and her daughter Talia Jansen had kindly invited me to The Greyhound of the Year Award dinner dance tonight. I took Mike Cooper and we had great fun. Debbie sat me next to the event chairman Maurice Watkins, a dynamic philanthropist who is also a serious Breakthrough Breast Cancer supporter. Interestingly, Maurice told me that the charity's researchers in Manchester had discovered that doctors could safely replace lymph glands taken from the underarm area with ones from elsewhere in the body, solving the current problems of oedema, etc, from multiple lymph gland removal. I remembered the Middle Eastern lady whom I had met at a party telling me how much she had suffered after having all her lymph glands removed 'just in case', and had had terrible discomfort and swelling for several months afterwards. This sounded like a huge breakthrough.

In the paper today there was an article by Tracy Somerset, the Marchioness of Worcester, who had had successful treatment for Stage 3 breast cancer in 2009 and is also under the excellent care of Professor Smith and Mr Gui at the Marsden. Tracy had had a mastectomy, chemo and radio, followed by Herceptin and had gone on the alkaline 'cancer diet' along with several natural supplements. So far she has had no recurrence of the cancer, thank goodness, although her doctors have given her a fifty per cent chance of it returning. She puts its non-return down to her healthy diet, although she admitted some people called it 'quackery'. If only they wouldn't – it is so unhelpful to cancer patients, and complementing medical treatment with a healthy lifestyle has got to be the way to go. Sadly there were a lot of unhelpful comments about the 'quackery' bit on the paper's website where I read it.

MONDAY 28TH JANUARY:
Duke University Research

Today there was an article in the Mail headlined 'Cancer patients who say No to a mastectomy more likely to survive'. Researchers from Duke University in North Carolina looked at the records of 112,154 women diagnosed with breast cancer between 1994 and 2004 and discovered that patients with early breast cancer actually stand a better chance of surviving the disease if they do *not* have a MX but instead have breast conservation surgery and radiotherapy. In fact women aged over fifty (the age when it seems to attack women most, I believe) who have only the lump removed, followed by radio, are almost a fifth more likely to survive than MX patients.

This is really interesting. If this information has been available since 2004, why have we not heard more about it before? I have always thought it is so much safer to have minor rather than major surgery. Plus there is the reconstruction to consider with a MX.

Only yesterday I heard from an older friend whose MX implant had disintegrated years later, requiring her to have major surgery once again, the poor thing. If you are slim and cannot use your own flesh for reconstruction, an implant is a necessity for aesthetic reasons. So the doctors are not just cutting the cancer out, but putting a foreign body in.

Once again I breathed a sigh of relief that friends and colleagues had advised me to have a second opinion about having a MX. I can understand that some former MX patients do not wish to hear this new information. But they have to take it on board in case, God forbid, they have a problem with their second breast, or their family or friends have to make a decision about which operation to have.

I feel quite strongly about this and feel another newspaper article coming on (I have been chronicling my case in the popular papers, trying to get my word out there. At least I have been proved right about the MX/lumpectomy debate. I had been 'trolled' online by women who said I would die if I did not have a MX, blah blah. Online trolls of professional women are sadly big news at the moment but hopefully the current feelings against them will curb this upsetting trend).

TUESDAY 29TH JANUARY:
Against Breast Cancer

Today I heard from Patricia Leathem, the Founder and a Director of the charity Against Breast Cancer. I had emailed her the *Daily Mail* article and she commented:

'As there are several types of breast cancer, mastectomy is sometimes the only option for some ladies. Also removal of only the lump means that some ladies would spend the rest of their life worrying that the cancer may return, so they choose mastectomy. So, as you say, the decision has to be left to the patient but with some guidance from the consultant regarding treatment.
'Our research is to stop this worry happening by preventing the secondary spread (cancer cells travelling to other parts of the body and ultimately killing the patient). Our aim is to

produce a vaccine that will be given to very young girls to
prevent the spread of breast cancer occurring.
'*We organise open days for our supporters to visit our labs at*
Westminster University to see and understand our research,
perhaps you would like to go to one of these open days?'

Pat's comments about the different types of breast cancer
and ladies fearing the return of the disease make perfect
sense. I do hope they produce the vaccine for young girls
soon. Sadly Jade and Kat are not young enough to benefit
from it. Thinking that both girls might have inherited the
breast cancer gene is one of my greatest fears. I am determined to visit ABC's labs asap.

In the afternoon, with my GP's OK, I had my first beauty
treatment since chemo and surgery, a Pelleve facial with the
fresh-faced (good advert!) Vicki Smith at Absolute Aes-
thetics. My face felt quite sensitive, possibly due to the
chemo, but looked much healthier afterwards and I treated
myself to a cup of tea and honey with dairy milk, in the
absence of soy!

Vicki and I discussed the latest *Mail* article with Dr
Kuldeep Minocha, the clinic's resident doctor, and he told
me I had done the right thing to get a second opinion and go
for the lump removal rather than MX.

ADVICE: Kuldeep advised me that, although radiotherapy is
obviously much easier to endure than chemo, I should still be
careful whilst on the course as it can affect different people in
different ways, and I must make sure to get plenty of rest.

FRIDAY 1ST FEBRUARY:
Blood Test For Dr Turner's Research (and drooping falsies!)

Now I have had surgery, including lymph gland removal on the left side, I can only have my blood taken from the right arm. This proved problematic today as my inner elbow veins refused to pop out and be injected and it was quite painful trying to get the needle in. The determined young male nurse said 'not to worry' and then tried one of my lower wrist veins which was successful but also quite uncomfortable (I later had a huge bruise and my wrist hurt when I signed cheques!). Tears sprang to my eyes – I am such a wimp! Then I thought about the poor tiger in a horrid TV advert by an animal charity (which should be banned, especially when kids are watching). The tiger had tears rolling down its so-human face and barbed wire around its neck and apparently later died. My little pinpricks were nothing compared to that and all the other horrible things that happen in this cruel world.

Luckily the serene Yukie from Research then appeared and made me feel better. She introduced me to breast nurse Nicky, who told me that my veins would be sore for a few months after chemo and that it was quite natural. We also discussed my current supplements and my fear of the possible side-effects of Tamoxifen and she said I would not have to have it if I did not want to – after all, I had had chemo as well as having radiotherapy.

Yesterday I read a newspaper article by Koo Stark, the first MX survivor I had thought of contacting when I had first been diagnosed. In the article she said she had resisted her talented hairdresser Neil Ward's suggestion to dye her hair after it went grey following her mastectomies and chemotherapy some years ago. Koo has always had beautiful hair and it looked gorgeous in a sort of steely grey colour. I can't imagine mine looking gorgeous if it turns out grey and I discussed this with staff nurse Elena, when I bumped into her today. She thought I had the right shaped face for short hair, however, so let's hope my little sprouts keep sprouting! Steven, my hairdresser, had brought round a new blonde wig cap for me as my previous one had become loose, encouraging wiggly 'slippage'. The new one is nice and tight but feels uncomfortable when I first put it on in the mornings. Oh well, no gain without pain – grow, grow, little sprouts!

In Koo's article she also mentioned that she had chosen not to reconstruct after her double mastectomy, the brave girl. However she had felt the need to wear a padded swimsuit when on holiday with her daughter and her daughter's friends (I can so understand that) and had bought a pricey one from a certain well-known shop. Apparently the falsies had become soggy and heavy when wet and drooped to her navel – yikes! What should unreconstructed mastectomy patients do? Try before you buy? Test the swimsuit in a bucket at the posh bra emporium? I had worn padded underpinnings from said shop for a play and found them very light – but I had not had to get wet! However this apparently happened to Koo ten years ago so let us hope the falsie manufacturers have got it sorted nowadays.

There was a picture of Michelle Heaton, the Liberty X singer, who had bravely had a double mastectomy and reconstruction when she heard that she had an extremely high chance of inheriting breast cancer, in yet another paper today (boob stories are everywhere these days!). She was showing off her reconstructed bosom and it looked amazing. Two different ladies, two different choices – it really is up to the patient.

SATURDAY 2ND FEBRUARY:
The Cost Of Rebuilding The Immune System

Poor Jeremy returned from The Nutri Centre today complaining about the cost of my antioxidant Co-Enzyme Q10 pills – £65 a bottle! I felt dreadful and immediately offered to repay him but he would not hear of it. So I asked my all-knowing nutritionist Peter Cox to explain the importance of these little gems.

ADVICE: Antioxidants are nutrients that 'mop up' oxygen free radicals produced during oxidative reactions. If not 'mopped up, these free radicals create oxidative stress or oxidation which damages tissue, including cell walls and cellular DNA. Oxidation is associated with damage that can trigger cancers, ageing and inflammation. In effect, oxidation is a by-product of respiring oxygen, like rusting. Antioxidants consumed within our food help slow the inevitable oxidation and afford us some protection against oxidative stress. Antioxidants can be divided into three groups: primary antioxidants (vitamins A, C, E), nutrients that are required for the synthesis of antioxidant enzymes (selenium, zinc, copper and manganese) and phytonutrients, such as resveratrol, xenoanxthins and cate-chins. Many nutrients have an antioxidant effect but these are considered the most important.

So now we know – keep taking the tablets!

SUNDAY 3RD FEBRUARY:
Sports Massage

Jade and I trotted off to The Hurlingham Club for sports massage, which I was ready for nearly two months after surgery and which proved very effective. The masseur, Marek, is also a physiotherapist who has treated several cancer patients and was very helpful, releasing my left shoulder and arm, which I had overstretched during my physio exercises. He also massaged all my muscles, which were aching a bit after my return to my regular tennis, cycling and weight training activities.

ADVICE: Marek told me to press down on my lymph scar and move the skin over it for a few seconds every time I applied the scar cream to stop any scar tissue building up. He also advised me to massage my scalp regularly, which apparently frees up the stress-holding neck and shoulder area. This is easy to do when you have no hair! Finally he suggested I add collagen supplements to my arsenal, to aid the connective tissue – oops, more expense – but you cannot put a price on good health, so I will investigate this suggestion.

That evening my husband, my brother and I attended

Mandie Adams Mcguire's fun quiz in aid of The David Adams Leukaemia Appeal for The Marsden. I cannot truthfully say that we won! However we met a lovely doctor and professor from the Marsden, Faith and Gareth, who told me I was in wonderful hands and on the home stretch now. They said I should not worry about my recent uncomfortable blood test: it was probably just a one-off with a young technician and Gareth said that he had once had a technician who had scraped the vein (not at the marvellous Marsden of course!)

TUESDAY 5TH FEBRUARY:
Run For Your Wife And Radiotherapy Tattoos

Rose-Marie and I tottered off to the premiere of Ray Cooney's funny film *Run For Your Wife*, which our mate Vicki Michelle had exec-produced. I wriggled into an underwired bra and plunging evening gown for the first time since surgery and felt that my dear little left boob looked much the same as before. Rose-Marie was wearing the exact same plunging evening gown and we had a huge laugh about it. Vicki and Annie Michelle (Jade's Godmum) and all their family were thrilled to see me out and about and kicking up my heels and I was thrilled to see them. I was also happy to meet Vicki's friend Ann – whom I had spoken to in my dark days in June – in the flesh. She had tragically lost her mum to breast cancer but survived herself after having an initial lumpectomy, then a third of her breast removed. Now, luckily, she is fine and we compared our little black

216

radiotherapy 'tattoos'. Ann had had her treatment several years ago so I guess it is true – radio tattoos really are permanent!

THURSDAY 7TH FEBRUARY:
First Radiotherapy Session, A Tan And A Party

What I was actually having was 'adjuvant external beam radiotherapy to left breast to complete breast conserving therapy'.

Jade knew I was nervous, as usual, and kindly came in with me, bless her. She was very surprised – as I had been the first time I visited 'radio' – when the small stairs near the Wallace Wing reception suddenly opened out to this huge area covering much of the basement level. The radiotherapy area comprises four units, we were told, and it is surprisingly light and airy for a basement, possibly because it is painted white, not green like many hospitals.

Jackie, the friendly receptionist, said, 'You *do* look alike' to Jade and me, which cheered me up hugely as my girl is just gorgeous! Then we went in to the little waiting room for the 'Lederman', the machine that would deliver the radiation. The radiotherapy area is for both private and NHS patients but, to my mind, the whole of the Marsden is like a private hospital, so perfect.

When my time came, Jade got up to come with me and hold my hand, as she always had for chemo but the nurses told her that she would not be allowed into the actual radiotherapy room – due, of course, to the radiotherapy! She looked at me with big frightened eyes and the kind nurses then invited her to have a look at the room so that she would at least know what it was like. She poked her head around the corner and presumably thought it was not too scary because she then pronounced it fit for mother, gave me a kiss and returned to the waiting room and her texting.

The room actually looked very space-age with various machines and screens around and everything painted white with dark blue trim. The radio ladies, Melissa, Lucy and Punita, were all sweet and relaxed me. I took off my top, donned the blue gown and lay down on the bed. They then drew bigger circles round my 'tattoo' dots and aligned me so that the beams would zap me in the right place. They placed my left arm up behind me into a holding device to keep it away from the 'zapping zone'. This was one of the reasons why Kate had given me the physio exercises after surgery to keep my arm and shoulder mobile so that I could easily raise the arm into this position. My gown was replaced after the marking of the tattoos as radio can zap through cotton.

Once lined up, the ladies left the room and told me to raise my right hand if I needed anything. When they left me alone I had a brief moment of panic. Other radio patients had said they had had some pain but not breast cancer patients so I was not really expecting to be hurt. But, me being me and a super wimp, I suddenly thought, 'What if something goes wrong and the machine drops on top of me and I can't get off the narrow bed?' A ridiculous thought at the safe-as-houses Marsden, of course, but a beauty thera-pist had once dropped a badly secured magnifying mirror on my nose during a facial so I am always nervous of any machine that is above me.

Latterly, whenever I have had a panic attack I have remembered the words of both of my psychics, Peter Lee and Valentin Borissov: 'You will have a long life' – and my new burlesque friend Fabia Cerra had recently read my palm and said the same thing. Nowadays of course I also have Lucien's self hypnosis technique to fall back on and can close my eyes and visualise myself in a beautiful place. So I lay back and thought not of England but of Atlantis in the Bahamas, where Jade and I one day want to swim with the dolphins. But I did not have a long mental sojourn in the Caribbean as the actual radiotherapy was so quick.

The treatment was of course completely painless and really quite relaxing. I thought I could feel a bit of warmth but I think that was probably just my over-active imagination working overtime again. There was a whirring sound when the machine, a Varian 'linear accelerator', zapped me from one side. Then it whirred more loudly as it rotated round my body to zap me from the other side. It is quite a big machine and as it rotated over me it reminded me of the spaceship coming over the hill in *Close Encounters Of The Third Kind*!

Then it was all over, just ten minutes after entering the Lederman suite, and Lucy asked if I had any questions. I didn't really – it had all been so quick and I had not felt a thing. The actual zapping probably only takes under a minute from each angle although it takes the nurses longer to manoeuvre you into the exact right position for the beams. Once in position you have to lie perfectly still, of course, but it's for such a short time that it's no hardship.

ADVICE: *Lucy said I could shower and bath normally but*

should not soak the area, not use too hot or very cold water and that I should use a bland, unscented soap. She told me to ditch the Youki (a new scar cream I was using after I ran out of Scarguard) on my bust whilst on radiotherapy but to use the aloe vera 99.9% gel which Marianne had advised me to use another lifetime ago and which I had duly bought in preparation for my big radio moment. She said to use it over the whole breast to ward off possible dryness and soreness.

When I looked at my phone I had an email from my hairdresser friend Neil Ward, whom I had emailed recently as Steven was away. I was a bit depressed about the darker, greyer, wirier feel of my hair sprouts but Neil wrote, 'When your hair comes back do not despair, it will grow out of the Brillo feel and look and, in my experience with clients, the hair will be 25% thicker'. Goodo, can't wait!

In the evening Vivien King-Lawless and I had a spray tan at The Village of Beauty. This was the first time I had literally bared my – slightly indented and still with a blue streak from the lymph gland dye – breast to anyone since my surgery but the nice salon owner, Kamilla, was very understanding so I guess my boob is acceptable. It certainly made me feel better to have some colour.

That night was Rose-Marie's very lively birthday party at her flat and I was very good, having only a mouthful of cake with no icing. A couple of people spoke to me about cancer. One lady had had a lumpectomy and chemo followed eventually by a MX and chemo and agreed that it was better to try the smaller operation first. She said that, after MX, they had put a large implant in, much bigger than her natural size, and she had had to have it removed and exchanged for a smaller one. She was really upbeat and positive but I felt sad about the extra unnecessary operation she had had to have on top of everything else. However she just said, 'There are so many worse things in life than breast cancer treatment' – what a star.

ADVICE: *Check with your surgeon about your implant(s) – size matters!*

Another person at the party, a chap, also told me about his mum, whom he had sadly lost to cancer recently. She had been given just five months to live but had actually survived for twelve years until last year. The human spirit is an amazing thing.

FRIDAY 8TH FEBRUARY:
Second Radiotherapy Treatment

Today I knew what to expect and was in and out very quickly. Two new – also very nice – ladies, Diana and Helen, had joined Lucy, and I just closed my eyes and relaxed. I can deal with this!

ADVICE: *You only have to take off your clothes in the area where you are being zapped – so, for breast cancer patients, just the top half. I now know to wear a claspless bra, which I roll down to my waist with my vest, and a zip-up cardy under my jacket. Thus I am in and out super fast. I guess the prostate guys lie there sans trousers, God bless them, but maybe they are allowed to keep their socks on!*

SUNDAY 10TH FEBRUARY:
First Effects Of Radiotherapy And The BAFTAs

After my second session, my breast started to feel a bit stingy and I could see a small red burn mark just on the edge of the scar on the aureole. I realise this is a particularly sensitive area due to both the position and the scar but, being me, I was very cautious. I immediately slathered my aloe vera 99.9% gel all over the breast, as instructed by Lucy, and went bra-less, which was more comfortable. The gel relieved the discomfort very quickly but I kept bras off for a couple of days, as even my soft sports bra rubbed the area.

Tonight was the BAFTA Film Awards and, being a loyal BAFTA voter, I wanted to look my best. Luckily I had been warned by radiologist Paolo that my usual underwired, padded bras might not be comfortable and Lucy had told me not to put anything on my lymph scar, which was still quite dark, being new – but I was prepared! Gill Harvey, Vivien's designer colleague at Medici, had kindly loaned me a gorgeous backless, low-cut white dress with sleeves. It was cut on the bias and skimmed me without constricting the bosom and the sleeves covered my scar.

Jade accompanied me and as we tottered up the red carpet on our vertiginous heels (in front of the gorgeous Eddie Redmayne, no less), it started snowing – this would never happen at the Oscars! At least my white dress blended in.

It was a magical evening in spite of the snow, with popular wins for Daniel Day Lewis and Juno Temple (both Old Bedalians like Jade), *Argo* and *Skyfall*, now the biggest grossing British film of all time, and most of the actors and films I voted for came in – I should have made some bets!

I later examined the Net photographs of the event with a magnifying glass and decided my bustline looked fine. A casual observer would never know I had just had a lumpectomy and 'lymphectomy'. Thanks again, Mr Gui.

MONDAY 11TH FEBRUARY:
Late For Treatment

Most of my radio treatments had been booked for 1.30pm but today's was at 12.50pm. However, I turned up at 1.30 after taking Jade to a casting and missed it! The staff were all very nice about it and fitted me in but I had to wait for a while, feeding the parking meter all the time, and I learnt my lesson. I was eventually treated in a different radio room, although it looked much the same and my *Close Encounter* was the same. I also had a male radiologist today called Ben – perhaps I was in the gents' side!

ADVICE: Never be late for your appointments if you can help it. The hospitals are busy and sadly there are loads of patients. In general the afternoons seem to be busier for most treatments.

The atmosphere was quite social in the little radiotherapy waiting room. One nice lady remembered she had modelled with me in the Seventies (we must have been in our prams!) She had had chemo and was now starting radio but had managed to avoid surgery, thank goodness.

Another jolly chap was there for prostate cancer. He said

he had had no surgery or chemo and was being treated by radio alone – brilliant. However he did say that the radiologists liked to treat the prostate patients with a full bladder, so that must be leg-crossing time if they have to wait too long! I told him that we women were not expected to have full lactating bazookas and we had a good laugh; I do hope I see him again, he cheered me up.

TUESDAY 12TH FEBRUARY:
Charing Cross Hospital Saved!

NHS North West London had been trying to close down most of the Charing Cross Hospital, particularly the excellent A&E department. We, the locals, had all been urged by the Council to 'resist' and sign petitions and put posters up, which our household had done. Today we heard that the hospital had been saved – a happy ending. I personally had had some scary times with a couple of the breast unit consultants there but most of the staff, their A&E Department and their Maggie's (Cancer Caring) Centre were all great.

Today I saw the nice chap in radio again. He told me that his brother was also being treated for prostate cancer, the poor man.

ADVICE: *If a blood member of your family has cancer, please get checked. Sadly there definitely seems to be a family connection. This is something that should be discussed with your doctor, because the number of affected family members and their age(s) at disease 'onset' are also important.*

I began to wonder if my grandparents had had cancer.

They had died before I was born but maybe cancer was not detected in those days. My parents had not had it although one of my uncles had got it late in life. Perhaps it can skip a generation. It is always worth looking into one's family health history to be safe.

Later I went to John Bell and Croyden for a promotional evening for their health and beauty products and luxuriated in a long Weleda foot massage. I had my collagen level read and it was very low, apparently lower than the previous person who was 70 years old! I know chemo dries the skin and maybe that affects one's collagen. (The next day I asked my GPs' surgery whether collagen supplements worked and they said there was no evidence to that effect. So, sorry, Marek at Hurlingham, I am not going to take anything at the moment unless it definitely works. My collagen may be low but my cancer has gone and that is my priority at present. If it *might* work and cannot harm me, I might try it in the future when I finally get off the ten supplements I am currently taking to rebuild my immune system.)

Then I met an old friend for a drink. He was amazed to see me looking well (thanks to Crystal and make-up) and told me he had been through it with his father. He remembered accompanying his dad to the hospital for his chemo treatments and seeing tears in his eyes from the pain. I would like to have known more about his father but was too upset to ask. There is no doubt in my mind that the family ('carers') of cancer patients suffer as much emotionally as the patients themselves. There is nothing worse than watching a loved one suffer, particularly when that loved one is your parent whom you have always looked up to and respected. I salute them all.

Remembering my own tears in front of poor Jade in the chemo unit I do not now feel so ashamed. God, I hate cancer and what it does to you. At the moment I am very weepy the whole time but put it down to lack of sleep and anxiety about the future. Lucien's hypnotherapy and the Melatonin spray seem to have cut down my insomnia but my sleep patterns are not yet perfect.

ADVICE: *Get plenty of rest while on radiotherapy. Apparently it drains you and the effects are cumulative.*

WEDNESDAY 13TH FEBRUARY:
End Of First Week Of Radio!

Today is the end of my first radiotherapy 'week' (comprising the five weekdays) so I am a quarter of the way through this, my last course of treatment! So far I have been treated in three separate rooms. The other two were not as pretty as my usual white and dark blue one but one of them, The Carlyle Suite, had a picture of waving palm trees on the ceiling above the bed so that, when the lights went on, you could look up and imagine being in the Caribbean!

I have had lots of different radiotherapists – Kay, Kieran, Faz, Rosemarie, Diana – all very pleasant in the usual Marsden way. I had noted in the doctors' letters, which I am still being copied in on, that they still describe me as 'pleasant'. I wonder if some patients are 'unpleasant'! Maybe if you had been told you were terminal you could be for-given for screaming and shouting a bit. In fact almost all the patients I have encountered at the hospital have been upbeat and positive (there was one rude old bat in radio but then there is always one, isn't there? Maybe I will be crabby when I am old and, God forbid, have to have treatment). On the whole, I think the general calm feeling of the Royal Marsden makes the patients calm.

Luckily I am not feeling too bad – a slight soreness throughout the whole breast but apparently this is normal and no recurrence of the slight burning on the actual skin surface. The nurses told me they monitor patients' skin closely and have various products to apply on anyone who goes especially red and sore. A girlfriend suggested honey gauze pads if I became especially sore and the aloe vera doesn't soothe it any more and apparently they stock these at the hospital for radio patients.

THURSDAY 14TH FEBRUARY:
Cancer-Causing Foods And Earliest Mammograms

After snow and rain all week, today was warmer with a pink and blue sky complete with fluffy clouds and intermittent sunshine. I visited Jo Miller, a long-time girlfriend and we walked her dogs on the common; it felt almost spring like – a bit like me, really. It seems as if I have been through a long hard winter and am now seeing some little rays of sun.

Jo, a former fitness guru, is very knowledgeable health wise and takes great care with her lifestyle and diet.

ADVICE: *We discussed an email she had just been sent:* 'WATCH WHAT YOU BUY. ESPECIALLY "HIGHLINER" FISH PRODUCTS; *they all come from China. Even though the* box says 'product of Canada', <u>it is from China</u> and 'processed' in Canada; that is, only the coating is added and packaged in Canada. The fish are raised in pens using chemicals that are banned in Canada as CANCER CAUSING but legal in China. This was exposed on CBC TV's Marketplace.'

This is quite ghastly and disgusting. Jo and I decided that it is always safest to buy fresh food from butchers, fishmongers and markets if you have the time, and that you must always read all food labels carefully if you shop at supermarkets. We decided that Waitrose was probably the safest in our local area.

Jo has two lovely daughters, film star Sienna and designer Savannah, and understood my worry about the possibility of Jade inheriting breast cancer from me and Kat inheriting it from her mum, Marilyn. She told me what her own doctor had said.

ADVICE: *Jo's doctor told her that young women could have efficient mammograms from the age of thirty-five. I had read that breast tissue is too dense to get a good reading until the age of fifty. When the time comes, get several opinions – ask everybody! Some people dislike mammograms because of the radiation but you will have a lot more radiation if, like me, you actually get breast cancer and have to have radiotherapy!*

FRIDAY 15TH FEBRUARY:
Fashion Week And Fake Nipples!

Jade was modelling at various London Fashion Week shows and one of my favourite 'walkers', Gino Chiappetta, accompanied me to watch her strut her stuff at the Rohmir show at Freemason's Hall. This is a huge great rabbit warren of a building with big rooms with high ceilings, perfect for fashion shows.

Jade loved working for Olga Roh, the glamorous Russian designer, and I loved looking at the gorgeous frocks and realising that I could wear most of them with my not-much-changed boob and tiny scars.

At the show I bumped into the actress Pauline Collins, whom I had not seen for ages, looking petite and pretty as a little deer. Pauline told me a funny story about a friend of hers who had had a mastectomy and reconstruction, but not the nipple adding bit. This lady had apparently bonded with her nice female surgeon and one day the surgeon rang her and said, 'Do come over, I have a present for you'. Then she gave her a fake nipple and said she would attach it for her! It is amazing what they can do nowadays.

I remember in my dark days turning down the nipple reconstruction idea as one operation too many and being criticised by my first, less than kind, surgeon. How important are nipples? I mused. Are they the cherries on the top of our Knickerbocker Glories? Would a loving partner miss one? Ultimately, ladies have to please them-selves but I have been told that the nipple operations are painless, which is one less thing to worry about. Certainly my aureole scar and radiotherapy to the area have not been painful, just slightly uncomfortable at one point.

SATURDAY 16TH FEBRUARY:
My Poor Neighbour Suffers With 'Chemo Veins'

My neighbour – who had been having chemo at the Marsden for several weeks after stomach cancer surgery – rang me in a terrible state. The poor girl said it had taken the nurses six goes to get a cannula into one of her veins last week and that she had been screaming in pain. Remembering what a state I had been in the day it had taken them four goes with me, I felt dreadful for her. She has had chemo every week for fifteen weeks. Frankly I am surprised that her poor veins are still taking it.

I had got thrombophlebitis in one of my big, back-of-arm veins just halfway through my course of eight and inquired about a PICC line and Port. Many other patients I know have suffered greatly in their chemo veins, particularly dear Billy Carter who put up with nine unsuccessful attempts at cannulation before stomping off to see the head of the hospital and demanding a Port (*not* at the Marsden!).

This lady, however, wanted to keep her treatment secret, so the line was not an option because the end of it (where the drugs are administered and blood taken) is attached to the arm and is visible, although covered with a bandage. She felt the Port, involving surgery to insert it, was too much with only five sessions to go.

She was already having the Lorazepam to calm her anxiety and they had plunged her arm in very hot water before cannulation, which I believe works better for numbing the discomfort of cannulation into smaller veins than anaesthetic gel, which shrinks the veins. Therefore the only advice I could give her was to wait for senior nurse Sophie, senior nurse Sally or nurse Valerie – the three nurses whom I remember as magical cannulators who could 'cannulate a brick'! I know there are patients who may be 'iller' but I do not think it is selfish to ask for a particular nurse if you have suffered the previous time. Plus it is upsetting for all the patients and nurses in the open-plan chemo area if a patient is actually crying or screaming, and the stress is very bad for the actual patient.

My neighbour also mentioned that many patients there were having secondary courses of chemo. Naturally this upset her but at least they would know what to expect, the poor things.

ADVICE: *I have said this before and I believe it is helpful to the hospitals as well as to the patients... If you are having a long course of chemo and/or your veins are not very prominent, inquire about a PICC Line or a Port. If, God forbid, I ever have to have chemo again in my life, I am fairly sure I would request one or the other and get all the stress over in one go. It may be extra work and expense initially for the hospital but it makes it so much easier for the busy chemo nurses as well as the patients in the long run. Remembering how good my surgery and anaesthesia were at the Marsden, I would not now be so fearful of the small operation to have a Port inserted.*

When I told Jade about our poor neighbour's cannulation problems she teared up just remembering the day it had happened to me.

MONDAY 18TH FEBRUARY:
Marking Up For My Boosters

After my treatment today I saw Dr Gillian Ross, the consultant clinical oncologist in Radiology, whom I had seen before starting my course. Dr Ross, a kind and reassuring lady has very long hair, which I envy!

She told me my skin was currently fine (maybe thanks to the aloe vera gel) and she and nurse Di marked me up for my 'booster' week at the end of my first three weeks of all-over (the breast) radiation. The booster treatment will be administered directly onto the 'tumour bed' – the site where the cancer was, rather than to the whole breast – thus the marking up.

In between my treatment and my consultation with the doctor I grabbed a sandwich in the Outpatients' Café and did a quick electronic questionnaire. I was pleased that the hospital was getting feedback on their cleanliness, punctuality, efficiency, communication and courtesy and was happy that I could give them very high marks in all areas.

TUESDAY 19TH FEBRUARY:
A Funeral And No Weddings

Today I went in to the hospital at 9am as I had to attend a funeral. It was so quiet at that time, with hardly anybody around and I was in and out very quickly.

ADVICE: *If you can bear to get up early, it always seems to be quieter in the mornings. The Marsden were very good about*

fitting me in when I wanted to come but I noticed that the
MDU where I had my chemo was also much quieter in the
morning.

After my treatment, my long-time friend from my
Hampshire days, Charlie ST, collected me and drove me
down to my home village for the funeral of our mutual
friend Nick. Nick was one of my few friends who had not
died of cancer but he was still gone too soon, may he rest in
peace.

It was a beautiful day for a send-off, cold but sunny with
a blue sky and fluffy clouds. The service was held in our old
church and it was a very emotional day for me, as both my
parents' funerals had been held there. The vicar told me that
Vicar Andy, who had presided in our day, had been pro-
moted but everything else looked the same. After the service
I placed a rosebush on my parent's graves in the leafy
churchyard. The one I had brought them last summer was
still going strong, so now my mother and father had one
each. I told them I would not be seeing them just yet after
all but that they would always be in my heart.

Then Charlie and I checked out my old house next to the
churchyard.

Every time I go back, the new owners seem to have
changed something else about it. We used to have a large,
rambling garden with lots of different flowers and trees. I
remember the Indian summer of 1991, when I sat in the
grassy garden with my parents, my back against our old oak
tree, my tummy huge with Jade. Now our old garden is a
gravel driveway with an ugly, modern six-car garage. As I
pressed my nose against the gate to get a better view of my

old bedroom, it suddenly swung open and I jumped back in alarm so Charlie and I quickly went on our way to the wake in the Church Hall.

I missed my parents and my old home terribly but I enjoyed catching up with the locals at the wake, who all wished me well with the rest of my treatment. Charlie stayed down in Hampshire on business, so his friendly daughter Naomi drove me back to London and my current life. We got caught up in bad traffic on the way back but it did not faze me as I am much more mellow these days – maybe from going through cancer, maybe from all the hypno and healing I have had.

WEDNESDAY 20TH FEBRUARY:
Shades Of Ouch And Some Good News For A Cancer Survivor

As I stretched my arm up into the restraint-type thing that holds your arm away from your bust during radiotherapy (very *Shades of Grey*!), I also stretched the breast and I felt a sudden pain inside, presumably at the tumour site. The nurses – Karen and Di today – assured me it was quite normal. They explained that the tissues were knitting back together after surgery and maybe did not like being bombarded with radio beams. But they were pleased that my skin is not too red, doubtless thanks to putting on aloe vera gel religiously twice a day, especially at night when senior staff nurse Edith had told me it would be particularly efficacious.

My friend who had had a lumpectomy and radio five years ago at the Sutton Marsden, and had been on Tamoxifen, rang to say she had had her five-year all clear! This was wonderful news, as the general understanding of cancer is that if it has not returned after five years it will not return at all. So huge congratulations were in the air. Hopefully she will now be able to come off Tamoxifen and lead a drug-free life. She said she had not had bad side-effects from it but had definitely put on weight, something which is always important to us ladies.

THURSDAY 21ST FEBRUARY:
New Tricks – 'Chemoradiation' – Chemo And Radio Together

As I wobbled off to the hospital today on Priscilla, my trusty bike, it started snowing. I had my thermals on and wasn't worried, as I have not caught a single cough or cold since Patricia Peat's cocktail of supplements kicked in.

While I sat in the little waiting room I saw two patients attached to drip stands. From the familiar clicking noise and the large cannulas, I deduced that they were chemo patients. I spoke to one of the ladies, Siobhan, who was accompanied by her sister Ellie, and she told me that she was indeed receiving chemo drugs at that very moment and would have a radio session whilst on them, as this 'chemoradiation' combination worked really well for her type of cancer, cervical. Siobhan was on a six-week radio course and would have chemo once a week for four sessions in the MDU. Then she would walk through the hospital with her drip for her radiotherapy and back again afterwards. She said that the drug she was on was Cisplatin, and that she did not really have bad side-effects with it.

While Siobhan had her treatment, Ellie told me that her

sister was only thirty and had been diagnosed after a smear test in October. By then it was apparently too late for surgery but she believed the chemo and radio combination would work well for her. Sadly the treatment would make her infertile but, thank God, she already had a fifteen-month-old daughter, Saoirse, and would focus on her.

Then Siobhan came out of the radiation room and showed me a photo of the adorable Saoirse. She seemed amazingly cheerful and upbeat and as the girls wandered back to MDU with the drip we said goodbye and wished each other well. An extraordinary young woman.

Later that day I spoke to Linda, the P.A. to Dr Gillian Ross and Dr Paolo De-Ieso, to check on some information about my case. Linda was charming and I told her how pleased I was with the all the staff and treatments at the Marsden. She said she was extremely touched, as no one ever said that. I was shocked and saddened to think that maybe these wonderful people were not appreciated enough.

ADVICE: If, like me, you have received excellent treatment at your hospital, do thank the staff. These guys do sterling work to keep us patients alive and healthy. I give my team little gifts of wine, chocolates and the occasional cake (after all they are not patients and are allowed these goodies!) but I believe words of thanks are just as important.

FRIDAY 22ND FEBRUARY:
Poets' Day And Physio

Funnily enough I was chatting to some patients in the waiting room today and we all agreed that the Marsden is beautifully decorated with a very calming atmosphere. One patient told us the story of a gentleman whose wife had sadly died in the hospital and he had donated a huge sum of money to get 'her' ward redecorated in bright cheerful colours – purple and giant flowers. Now that is real gratitude.

As I left the radiotherapy department today Jackie, the jolly receptionist who reminds me of the comedy actress Kathy Burke, said, 'It's POETS' Day today.'

'What's that?' I said naively.

'P off early, tomorrow's Saturday,' chuckled Jackie. I am so going to miss this jolly lot and can understand why some patients get very depressed when they finish their treatment and do not have to come to the hospital regularly any more. I will definitely pop in from time to time to say hello in their quiet times.

Today I had a consultation with my Marsden physio, clinical specialist physiotherapist Kate Jones, as my shoulder was still uncomfortable. The gentle Kate examined me and told me that it was probably just the combination of the surgery, overdoing the original physio exercises and now the radiation, which was upsetting my shoulder. However she gave me some new exercises for my shoulder muscles and said I would be able to go skiing, which was great news as Jeremy was very keen for us to have our usual family skiing holiday in March and visit Allie, his son who was working in Verbier. The bad news for Jeremy is that Kate advised me to ask him to carry my skis for me, just in case!

When I got home our financial advisor arrived to advise me about making a will. He also advised me to rethink some of my investments. When I was working regularly I was not too bothered about my savings but if, like me, you cannot do your usual work whilst ill you need to make your investments work for you, so look around for the best financial deals. If you are not going to work and even if you are in bed, you will be able to check the Internet, ring round the financial institutions and talk to advisors on the phone.

ADVICE: *If you have cancer it is only sensible to make a will to protect your family.*

SATURDAY 23RD FEBRUARY:
Rowena's Cancer Stories

My local friend Rowena Chowdrey popped round to see me. She is a photographer who really knows faces so I revealed my sprouting barnet to her. She said short hair would really suit me, which is good because it will be a long time short! Rowena cited Anne Hathaway and Dame Judi Dench as ladies she had snapped who looked great with a 'shorty'. Those beautiful women will be my inspiration when the time comes.

Rowena gave me an update about her friend Vicky who had recovered from a mastectomy a few years ago. Sadly cancer had returned in Vicky's neck and her liver. However she had been given an amazing new treatment, as yet unavailable on the NHS, which she thought was working. It had cost £50,000 but Vicky sensibly had health insurance.

ADVICE: *Take out health insurance early, long before you get sick if you can afford it. Remembering my problems with PPP* and my parents being badly misinformed by BUPA, I advise you to shop around.

Rowena also told me a harrowing story about a cancer patient she had befriended in our local hospital. Rowena had gone into A&E for a gallstone, which she had later happily passed, and been placed in a cancer ward as the hospital was full. The lady in the next bed had not been diagnosed with breast cancer in good time at her local hospital in the country, even though she was a nurse and felt sure something was wrong. Eventually she <u>had</u> been diagnosed and the surgeon had decided to give her a lumpectomy rather than a MX, saying 'that is what women prefer' and without discussing her case with her or giving her any options.

Tragically the lumpectomy had been too little, too late. The lady had transferred to the London hospital and had a mastectomy but by then the cancer had spread and later she tragically died. Before she died, however, she took the original surgeon to court for negligence, attending the High Court hearing in her wheelchair. The surgeon was not keen to answer questions and said to the judge, 'Don't you know who I am?' (shades of Alec Baldwin's pompous surgeon in *Malice*!)

The judge of course found for the tragic woman and that case set a precedent: patients should be given all the facts and all the choices available to them. High and mighty surgeons should not play fast and loose with their patients' lives.

ADVICE: *I am sorry to have to repeat this but it is so important to get a second opinion. I believe from my own* experience that you can get a second opinion from another surgeon in the same hospital (at least, that is what the original surgeon I saw at my local hospital told me) so it should not take too long and may save your life.

MONDAY 25TH FEBRUARY:
Meeting The 'Against Breast Cancer' Team

After my treatment today I finally met up with Pat Leathem and Wendy Taylor Hill from Against Breast Cancer and later with Dr Miriam Dwek, senior lecturer in biochemistry at the University of Westminster. Against Breast Cancer funds research taking place at Westminster University to prevent the spread of breast cancer to other parts of the body. Their ultimate aim is to produce a vaccine that will be given to young girls (pre-puberty) so preventing breast cancer. What a wonderful world that would be! I was thrilled when the kind ladies asked me to be a patron of the charity and just hope I can help them enough. They told me that their other patrons included Simon Cowell and his mum Julie, a former breast cancer sufferer who is also President of ABC, former Olympian Suzanne Dando and presenter Ben Shephard so I will have to pull my socks up!

I asked Pat, a former theatre nurse who is married to a doctor specialising in breast cancer, Wendy and Miriam several questions and they were all very helpful. They said that Tamoxifen is a wonderful drug so, if Professor Smith thinks it will work for me when the time comes, I will definitely have to try it.

ADVICE: The good news is that beer, containing hops, is good for cancer patients as the hops react against any stray cancer cells (and there was me feeling guilty for having a lager at the local pub recently when there was no decent red wine!). The ladies also said I should not stress about sticking religiously to the famous cancer diet – sugar and fats are not going to kill you (at least from cancer. Heart disease, maybe!) – and if you eat red meat twice a week rather than once it will help increase your haemoglobin and boost your immunity. In general, experts Pat and Miriam feel that, as with everything in life, 'moderation is the key' but they are currently conducting trials on diet and lifestyle for breast cancer patients and will have the definitive advice for us all very soon. This was music to my ears, as different nutritionists, health experts and authors 'out there' say different things about what is good and what is bad to eat for cancer and it is extremely confusing.

TUESDAY 26TH FEBRUARY:
Cancers Of The Sacrum, Ankle And Throat

My friend with cancer of the sacrum rang me today and told me that he was sadly getting worse, and less mobile. The knowledgeable Patricia Peat had put him in touch with top cancer specialist Professor Vogl in Germany. The professor had had considerable success working with soft tissue but not yet with bony tissue. I also put him in touch with 'bionic' Janie Martel, who suggested another specialist in Switzerland. Then we both tried to track down my bowel cancer friend Christine who had told me about the clinic in Dallas which 'guarantees' curing any cancer.

My friend says his cancer will not kill him but that, if it progresses without a halt, the side-effects of immobility, impotence, incontinence, colostomy bag, etc, would make his life not worth living and he was again talking about going to Dignitas to end it all. I felt dreadful for him but he is bravely fighting on and gave me the following advice – for all patients with cancer in their system.

ADVICE: Dr Michael Mosley has written a book called The Fast Diet *where he suggests patients eat only one quarter of their normal food intake on one day of the week. Apparently this tricks the cells into thinking they are being starved all the time and they regenerate. My friend has started the regime and believes that his cancer cells will die and be reborn as healthy cells. If it works it would be wonderful – certainly worth trying if you are as sick as him.*

Later I went to Kamini for some threading (now that my brows and moustache have returned!) and healing. Interestingly Kami said that my brow and upper lip hairs, like my lashes, have grown back in exactly the same pattern as previously, unlike my head hair which is darker, greyer and fuzzier, and my nails, which are much longer than before. Once Kami had threaded and dyed them, the brows looked nice and healthy again and I nodded off during her relaxing healing session.

Once finished I chatted to Natasha, Kami's receptionist, about my happy recovery. Natasha told me that she had recently been touched twice by cancer. Her little nephew had been diagnosed with bone cancer at the age of two. The poor little mite had had to have chemo and surgery to his ankle but the treatment had been entirely successful and now, aged six, he was running around happily.

Her partner Bruce had not been so lucky. He had had throat cancer, diagnosed late, and had suffered greatly from chemo and radio (apparently it is not pain free in the throat area), being unable to eat or drink and on a nasal drip. Natasha had stopped working and cared for him but Bruce had sadly passed away in November. When Natasha told me this I burst into tears – I felt so guilty wittering on about my successful treatment when *her* partner had died. Natasha hugged me and said, 'It's OK,' but it is not and never will be until we cure this dreadful disease which Natasha rightly calls 'the modern plague.'

I went home more than ever resolved to help with cancer research in any small way I can and started planning a small fundraiser for Against Breast Cancer – at least I can help the fight against my own type of cancer.

WEDNESDAY 27TH FEBRUARY:
Being Positive And Further Checks After Cancer

Today at the hospital I was treated in the LA3 radio suite, as the Lederman was being maintained. It is not as pretty and there are no palm tree patterns on the ceiling as there are in the Carlyle suite but I am still having my spaceship moment, which I have come to rather enjoy.

The beautiful Siobhan was there again, having just

radiotherapy today, with her mum Patricia and baby Saiorse, who is adorable. I can so understand why Siobhan wants to keep going and be positive for her little one.

ADVICE: *Dr John Keet reminded me to have a PET/CT scan at some point after completion of treatments to check my whole body and also mentioned genomics and proteomics. It is all Greek to me but I will check with Professor Smith when the time comes.*

THURSDAY 28TH FEBRUARY:
First Booster – And Party Time

Back to LA3 today and new tricks. The nurses placed me on the bed with a couple of blue foam pads behind my left side to wedge me into position. Then they got the tracing paper out and recreated the circle round my tumour area that Dr Gillian had marked last week. They had taken a photo of the doctor's markings and I was amazed at how good my famous Left Boob looked in the photo when my arm was behind my head and the breast was stretched (very Joan Collins in *The Stud!*)

ADVICE: *The girls carefully got me into position for my close up with the linear accelerator; the LA was very close but not touching, of course. I was a bit nervous at the proximity of the machine and advise patients to shut their eyes. As with the previous treatments, I could not feel anything and it was actually quicker this time as the booster only zaps the tumour area from the one angle. So no spaceships over the hill this time! In fact the actual zapping only takes about twenty seconds, nurse Kay told me, but it feels longer while you are lying there keeping your arm out of the way (no Shades Of Grey arm support with the booster treatment, so it is important to keep your arm and shoulder mobile with the physio exercises).*

When I asked how long each zap is with normal radio the nurses explained that the *dose* is always the same but the time the machines take to deliver it may vary slightly. It is only a matter of seconds for each dose though, usually well under a minute.

That evening I was taking Jade to a couple of dos and wanted to look my best in a low-cut dress Adele had given me. I had been advised not to wear underwired bras too often whilst having radiotherapy to the breast, so I unthreaded the wire bit from the left side of an otherwise soft-ish bra and put that on. My eyelashes were now long enough for me to wear mascara, rather than false lashes, for the first time – another small triumph along the road to looks recovery.

ADVICE: I am using the Revitalash nourishing mascara that my friend Angela Egan kindly sent me when she first heard of my 'hairless' problems, so that the lashes are actually being treated whilst fluttering once more.

The first event was a speech and book signing by the interesting thriller writer Ruth Rendell at the Mayfair Library. As I bent over so that the seated Ms Rendell could sign a book for Jade, I noticed Marilyn, the lady who had invited me, peering intently at my bazookas! Well, that is par for the course when people know you have had breast cancer surgery; if they cannot tell which breast was operated on, you must congratulate your surgeon. One of my black radio tattoos was clearly visible in my cleavage but so what? At least I still *have* a cleavage.

The next event was the launch of the new Intercontinental Westminster Hotel. Jade and I had been invited by our commercials agent, Vicki Field, and her husband Mark, the MP for Westminster. Vicki looked splendid, and we bumped into all sorts of other old friends. Everyone congratulated me on being nearly finished with everything and still looking like myself. I am always amazed at how people are fooled by Crystal – 'Oh, so you haven't lost your hair, then?' The received knowledge is that NHS wigs are rubbish but that is so not true, at least at the Marsden where Paul and Gill had offered me a huge selection of wigs by various manufacturers. Crystal is made by Natural Image but I have seen all sorts of gorgeous wigs on Marsden patients. If a male patient loses his hair, it is acceptable for him to have a shaved head because it is a certain 'style', but women need to have a choice: 'to hair or not to hair'. Crystal was now several months old and I had visited Paul earlier in the week to ask some questions on maintaining the wig.

ADVICE: *Paul advised me to use a wig brush to brush out any tangles caused by the wig rubbing against collars at the back and to style it and I found a nice one for £5-odd at Trendco in High Street Kensington. He also showed me how to attach the welts of the wig on to the wig cap with grips to secure it. (Now that my own hair was growing a bit, the spirit gum I had been* using to attach the cap to my bald head was sticking to my tiny new hairs and I did not want to lose any of the precious little things!) Paul told me a salutary tale about a patient who had chosen a wig from him and proceeded to glue Velcro strips to her scalp and Velcro the wig, in spite of him telling her not to. Sadly she got some nasty sores on her head that became infected – horrid.

FRIDAY 1ST MARCH:
Siobhan's Bravery, And 'Chemo Feet' at La Durbin

This morning I saw Kate in physio and she told me my shoulder was recovering well with the new exercises she had given me. So full steam ahead for skiing!

Siobhan was back in Radiotherapy with her last chemo drip today and her sister Ellie. She had unfortunately got a nasty vomiting bug for a couple of days and had to miss chemo yesterday. As she got up to go to her treatment I noticed she was very slim and Ellie said that she had lost much of her appetite and seven kilos in weight. But she was as upbeat as ever. The girls told me that, after finishing her normal radio course next week, Siobhan would then have brachytherapy: radiation where the dose is given through rods internally. She will have to keep completely still for two whole days, so will be admitted to hospital where they will insert the rods during anaesthesia and she will have to have a catheter as well. It is the final stage of her treatment for cervical cancer, administering a localised higher dose of radiation. I guess it is the equivalent to my booster for breast cancer.

I gulped when I heard all about the treatment, which sounds very hard, but managed to paste a bright smile onto my face for Siobhan's sake. She is being so incredibly brave and I know she is doing it all for her family, especially her dear little Saiorse. They are obviously a very close family and come up to the hospital every day on the train and tube from Croydon. I so hope she will be completely cured with all this treatment.

That evening Charlotte and I attended the opening of La Durbin, a new beauty salon in our area. The friendly owner, Latifa, suggested I have a pedicure but I was a bit shy about showing my feet, which had become dry and scaly and my toenails broken and flaky during chemo. However, kind beautician Lana assured me they are in fact very healthy now, which is a huge relief as, at one stage, I was worried the toenails might actually fall off. I certainly felt much better after Lana's nice massaging and with some 'Breast Cancer Pink' polish on my toenails. It seems that all of my external bits are now growing nicely – I just hope that my immune system and my cells inside are also doing the business.

SATURDAY 2ND MARCH:
Ellie, Lorraine And Carol – Cancer Is All Around Us

As I had not been able to work much while ill, I had got used to not wearing make-up and become lazy about putting it on when I was going out. So I had decided to treat myself to some Permanent Make Up on my eyelids and lips after my radio finishes. The expert I had chosen was Tracie Giles, who was represented by my pal Lucy Dartford. Tracie knew my story and told me about her brave young niece Ellie Sedgwick, who had sadly got cancer when she was just 16. Today I spoke to Ellie on the phone.

Ellie told me that she had had Hodgkin's Lymphoma, Lymphocyte Predominant, a cancer which attacks the lymph nodes. She said that in 2010 when she was just 16, she had noticed a largish lump under her jaw. However it did not really show much and her mum thought it was probably just a bad reaction to having her ears pierced when she was run down, what with studying for exams, etc.

However it gradually grew bigger so in 2011, when Ellie was 17, she went to her GP but her blood tests appeared normal. She was then referred to her local hospital at Bury St Edmunds, where she was given a needle biopsy and an ultrasound and they found seven lumps in her neck and had to perform a full biopsy on her big lump, which was sadly malignant.

At this stage Ellie was referred to Addenbrooke's Hospital in Cambridge where they performed a PET/CT Scan and discovered the cancer had spread to her sternum and abdomen, making it Stage 3. The hospital put her on a seven-month course of chemo, firstly on a regime called ABVD, which was unsuccessful, then R-CHOP, which happily worked very quickly and got rid of the tumours completely.

Ellie said her side-effects were not too bad, no vomiting and no real nausea, just a bad taste in the mouth, lots of painful unpleasant mouth ulcers and extreme fatigue. However, her hair was affected and she decided to shave it all off early on. Her close school friends were very under-standing, however a lot of people didn't know how to react to someone who had cancer, especially at such a young age. Ellie stopped going to school due to feeling so fatigued and focused on getting well.

She also lost all her lashes and brows but was luckily able to turn to her lovely 'Aunty Tracie' for Permanent Make Up, which made her feel much more human, she said. She was supported by the Teenage And Young Adult Unit at the hospital and said she made some amazing friends there. She has since become an Ambassador for The Teenage Cancer Trust, which supports the Unit.

By 2012 Ellie was luckily able to go back to school and get on with her life. She is now, at 18, studying for her A Levels, after which she will do a gap year, uni, and then she hopes to work for a cancer charity. What a totally amazing and inspirational young girl.

Talking to Ellie, who is forty years younger than me but so intelligent and mature and has been through so much, made me feel very humble. Ellie told me that she believes if she had known about the signs and symptoms of cancer, she would have gone to the GP sooner, which may have changed her experiences but who really thinks that they will get cancer at 16? I really enjoyed talking to Ellie and we wished each other well for the future.

Later I read an article in the paper about national treasure and actress Lorraine Chase, who has just admitted that she has whipped cancer twice, God bless her. Lorraine apparently had cervical cancer, treated successfully by laser, twelve years ago, and had had a carcinoma removed from her face just four weeks ago. Plus she cared for her long-time boyfriend John, who sadly passed away from lymphoma in 1996. She is so brave. I had invited her to my Yes To Life party in November and she never breathed a word about all her own problems.

Lorraine was quoted in the paper as saying she now intended to achieve her 'bucket list' of things to do before you die and that, if the cancer came back she would have a massive party then end it all at Dignitas. A photo of Dignitas I saw online did not look very appealing and knowing what I now know about chemo and how you can get through it so much more easily, I would encourage Lorraine or anyone whose cancer came back to try chemo before giving up. Sadly my friend with cancer of the sacrum is unable to have chemo but who knows what marvellous new cures they will find in the future? Lorraine is only sixty-one, which is not that old by cancer standards, so I sent her a message saying we all expected her to live a 'long, long, long' life. We cannot lose her, she is a fun, intelligent and highly principled lady.

While shopping at Tesco (my personal weekly nightmare and even harder now that I have less energy), I received a call from Carol Rodgers, a very intelligent American TV producer I had met through Dominick Mereworth. I updated her on my case and she told me that her mum had had breast cancer in her seventies and after treatment had been put on Tamoxifen for five years. Carol said that in the States they automatically put *all* breast cancer patients on to Tamoxifen and then on another drug for a further two years to wean them off Tamoxifen! They are certainly into preventative medicine in the States. Happily Carol's mum has just finished her seven years of drugs and is feeling great.

ADVICE: *Carol said that both her mum and her dad each eat three almonds a day, which is supposed to be a cancer preventative, and that they are both amazingly healthy in their eighties. I have heard about almonds for cancer before and am currently drinking almond milk (there are varying stories about both dairy and even soy milk vis-à-vis cancer.)*

As I was near the nuts aisle in the supermarket at the time I decided to substitute the usual family bag of peanuts for almonds. I wonder if the family will like them? They taste delicious and no one seems quite sure at the moment whether peanuts are a good anti-cancer food or not, although walnuts apparently *are*.

MONDAY 4TH MARCH:
Rash Time

As I re-read the title of my last chapter I could not help singing to myself 'Cancer is all around us – and so the feelings show' (with sincere apologies to Bill Nighy and *Love Actually*). I think I am losing it but you have to get some laughs out of this whole gruesome business. Mother Rytasha is still sending me her funnies regularly and they are keeping me sane.

Lorraine Chase messaged me back that 'we are made of good stock and just get on with it'. She is such a brave, positive lady. I have never felt particularly brave and am in fact terrified of death, in spite of my religious faith – but perhaps that gives you an edge when you are fighting such a deadly disease as cancer!

Over the weekend I had developed an itchy red rash on the top and underside of My Left Boob and desperately hoped I was not going to fall at the final fence with some nasty infection. However, Kay and the girls in the department assured me that it was quite normal, just a delayed reaction to my normal radio. Now that the booster was just zapping the one small area at the left of the breast above the tumour site, rather than all over as before, the rash area would not be attacked further.

ADVICE: RADIOTHERAPY RASHES 1. The nurses told me to keep applying the aloe vera gel, which is very soothing, and they would get me an appointment with the senior staff nurse tomorrow. They told me not to scratch the rash area as that would break the skin and make it worse. As the rash is itchy and scratching with my – now huge and talon-like – nails would break the skin, I will also wear soft cotton gloves at night. However the aloe vera is calming the itchiness for the moment.

This evening I watched a new BBC show called *Bang Goes The Theory*. The subject was plastic. For a long time I had been receiving emails advising me not to leave plastic bottles in my car in the sun and drink from them afterwards as, they say, an 'altered state' (melted) plastic bottle might leach into the water and potentially cause cancer, so I had been wary of plastic for a while.

However this programme informed the public that not only was it safe to drink mineral water from plastic bottles, but that it was also safe to use the bottles again. It also said plastic wrapping on food was safe. It touched upon a new study which suggested that environmental factors were involved in the rise of 'reproductive' cancers – breast and prostate – but did not tell us exactly which environmental factors.

So – we draw our own conclusions. Personally I am sticking to my water filter at home and buying glass instead of plastic bottles of mineral water where possible but I am not going to obsess about it.

TUESDAY 5TH MARCH:
Rashes And Cracked Lips

Today I bumped into my prostate cancer pal whose name, I have discovered, is Mark and his elegant wife Pat. They had just been to lunch at Le Columbier across the road and Mark confided that he had not exactly stuck to the 'Cancer Diet' today! But he did say that he had given up alcohol for quite some time after being diagnosed and only drank red wine very occasionally now as a special treat, so I was full of admiration for that feat. I am really going to miss all these lovely people when I finish my treatment tomorrow. Mark had finished today, hence the celebration.

After my treatment I had a consultation with the senior staff nurse to talk about my rash. I was delighted to see that the wonderful senior staff nurse Orla was on duty today. I had not seen her since my pre-surgery days with Mr Gui. It seems only yesterday that Jade and I were crying in Mr Gui's consulting rooms and Orla was comforting us. I had been very ashamed of my snivelling then but there have been many more tears since – and laughs. I guess Orla has seen it all. It is amazing how quickly my time as a cancer patient has gone by. It was a year ago that I had the fateful mammogram that would seal my fate – and eight months ago when I first started anti-cancer treatment.

ADVICE: RADIOTHERAPY RASHES 2. Orla gave me some hydrocortisone cream for the rash area and aqueous cream to keep the rest of the breast moisturised. She advised that any radio side-effects, such as my rash, would get worse for a couple of weeks after treatment before getting better and told me to put the creams on two or three times a day.

ADVICE: MOUTH CRACKS AND WOUNDS. I also spoke to Orla about my mouth, which had been very sore and cracked ever since chemo (definitely no kissing at the moment!). It had got to the stage where topical creams were not healing it any more and Orla suggested that I get some Lysine tablets from Holland and Barrett (I-Lysine,1000mg), which would heal the whole mouth area. She said it was just a low immune system problem and quite normal. I had also found that drinking through a straw was more comfortable and that leaving lipstick off and just using Lipsalve and Vaseline helped.

Nigel Dean, my travel agent pal, had sorted out our skiing holiday in Verbier to visit Allie, my stepson, and we were off in two weeks' time. I still get quite breathless on my bike after all my treatments and surgery so I am not planning any downhill racing!

However I did stop off at a sports shop called Altimus in High Street Kensington to buy a skiing helmet – going through what I have been through has made me much more protective of my life. I think I look like a complete plonker in the helmet but there is no point suffering through cancer treatments for several months then bashing your head in an unguarded instant on the piste!

WEDNESDAY 6TH MARCH:
Last Day Of Radiotherapy – Last Day Of Cancer Treatment! Tamoxifen Or Not?

Ben and Maxine looked after me today in LA3 and I was happy to report that the hydrocortisone was helping my itchy rash and that I had bought the I-Lysine tablets for my mouth problem. I felt rather sad when Ben announced, 'And now for your last radiotherapy treatment'. I hope I will see them all again but hopefully not for treatment! As I said before, I can so understand why patients become depressed and insecure after finishing long treatments, especially when they have got used to visiting the hospital every day – you are the centre of attention as a cancer patient and suddenly it is all over and you are a civilian once again. They are all so efficient in radio, always letting you know when they are running late, etc. If only Real Life was like that...

But this is not goodbye to the marvellous Marsden, where I have always felt so nurtured and protected; it is just 'au revoir'. I would be having another physio session with Kate before my ski trip, a check up with Mr Gui in July and I also had a long talk with the knowledgeable Geraldine, Professor Smith's PA, about my future vis-à-vis medication. Geraldine told me that they had analysed my stray cells after surgery and that the oestrogen reading was 6 out of 8 (as opposed to 3 out of 8 previously), which apparently meant that I <u>might</u>, after all, respond to Tamoxifen. She said that these sort of readings were not always as accurate as the original histology but that I should see the Prof asap because, if I did go on Tamoxifen, I should start sooner rather than later. So she made an appointment for me for the week after my skiing trip.

I have always been a little wary of Tamoxifen because so many of my friends said that they had had bad side-effects while on it and I believe it is a lengthy five-year course. More importantly, however, everyone I know who has been on the drug has had no recurrence of their cancer, which is the main thing. I think that if you can get through chemo and come out the other end with your sense of humour still intact, then you are pretty well equipped to deal with side-effects in the future. Many women put on weight, which is of course upsetting for us ladies, but perhaps it is then time to treat ourselves to some new frocks after all we have been through!

In the afternoon many friends rang to wish me well at the end of all my treatments. One was my theatrical agent, Rob Groves, whose dad had also just finished a course of radio the day before with no ill effects happily. Then my old flatmate, Debra Witt, rang to suggest a celebration soon and I am certainly up for that! Our friendly cleaner 'Sally 2' smiled happily for me as I answered all the calls.

Next up was 'bionic' Billy Carter, who is brilliant at tracking down new cancer cures. Billy said that in Japan and the Far East cancer doctors are now putting patients on AHCC, a completely natural cure made of different kinds of mushrooms, including the maitake mushroom, which Patricia Peat had recommended along with my other supplements. Billy had already ordered huge quantities from the Net, he said. Apparently AHCC has no side-effects and I will definitely check it out with Patricia and with the Prof at my upcoming consultation.

NHS patient Billy also said that he had persuaded his hospital to give him a PET/CT scan (which my doctor pals Anna Brocklebank and John Keet had suggested I have after all my treatments were over). He said the scan cost £1,500 so I guess I had better start saving up! It is fair for someone who has suffered as much as Billy to get a freebie on the NHS but I am officially well now and will have to go privately, I imagine.

Jade was on a shoot and Jeremy was in the office but we all met later on for a family dinner to celebrate. We chose Da Mario, our old haunt on Queensgate Terrace, where Jade had started her life. Naughtily I ate a creamy pasta containing both wheat and dairy but I thought I deserved a little treat on this night of nights. I vividly remembered sitting in that restaurant with Marilyn, Kat's mum, at least eighteen years ago when she was on Tamoxifen, recovering from her lumpectomy and clutching an alcohol free Kaliber lager as she had been told not to drink. How lucky breast cancer patients are today, I thought, being able to cheer ourselves up with alcohol, as I guzzled a fruity red wine! I have cut down and changed from white to red wine and will drink more lager (now that Pat Leathem has explained that it is good for mopping up stray cancer cells) but I do not think I could give up alcohol completely like some brave patients, especially with stomach cancer, have to do. My heart goes out to everyone who has to give up the things they love in life on account of their health.

THURSDAY 7TH MARCH:
Life Goes On After Cancer – And Always Do Your Best

Life goes on after cancer and today I had a meeting with my dynamic commercials agent Vicki Field, who introduced me to the equally dynamic David Samuels, who would handle TV bookings for me – should I get any! I do not know how producers and bookers react to artistes who have had cancer, regarding insurance and so on, but I guess I will find out. David mentioned reality shows and asked me if there is anything I would not do – I cannot imagine having the energy to dance, skate or dive from the high board but I told him I would always do my best at whatever came up.

That evening Tory supporter Stanley Holmes escorted me to the glitzy Conservative Party Spring Dinner at the Wyndham Grand Hotel in Chelsea Harbour. I wore a high-necked dress with no bra, which was comfortable and covered my rash, and tucked in to healthy fish, which I am now starting to enjoy. The guest of honour was the brilliant Julian (Lord) Fellowes, who was interviewed by Simon Heffer, and I laughed uproariously. Julian mentioned several times 'always doing one's best', which seems to be the Thought for the Day.

Various old friends – Tatiana, Sandra and Maggie – were on the table and wished me well. Another friend, Vivien, had had a successful mastectomy with the Marsden dream team of Smith And Gui eight years ago and was now happily in the rudest of health and wearing a pretty low-cut dress. With friendly companions, good food on my plate and a fruity red wine in my hand, it was good to be alive.

SUNDAY 10TH MARCH:
Mother's Day

Our dear girls Kat and Jade gave me beautiful cards, flowers and gifts for Mother's Day, then Jade made me a healthy salmon and juice lunch. I felt very spoiled and lucky.

In the paper today there was an article about the first lady to have chemo from a mobile NHS unit in the car park of her local Tesco – brilliant. These units will so help patients who live a long way from their hospitals. I hope there will be radiotherapy units soon too.

My NYC friend Iris Rossi had put me in touch with her breast cancer survivor friend Meredith Gray and today I watched a video of Meredith's 'Naked Project' on the Net. An inspirational lady who is helping other patients all over the world through her website.

Hopefully I will get to New York this year to see one of my best girlfriends, Robin Brand. Robin survived a hurricane last year and now I have survived cancer! Then I could visit my old mate Steve in Palm Springs, and then my friends Patrick and Annabel Curtis in Utah – now is the time for me to think about doing things I want to do rather than those that I have to do.

In the evening Jeremy took us out to dinner at our local Ta Krai Thai restaurant and I ate healthy stir-fried prawns and vegetables and tried a Singha lager, which was delicious. I cannot believe lager is actually good for cancer – what luck!

In general I am feeling pretty good. I suppose I am now in what is called 'remission'. My left boob appears slightly swollen and the rash is still itchy but those are minor considerations. I am working on my recurred mild insomnia with the melatonin spray and will have sessions with hypnotherapist Lucien Morgan and healer David Goodman soon. At least I am catching up with the Dean Koontz novels Jade gave me for Christmas if I cannot sleep. My anxiety dream of packing is back but I believe that is just the – quite normal – fear of returning to the real world after being cocooned in hospital life for several months.

My hair is at last growing back all over my head. It seems to be thicker than before and is now looking blonder, more like its original colour. Jeremy says it feels like a mat – or maybe he meant 'matte'! My husband is not much given to compliments but he did say I was not a hypochondriac and had 'got through everything' very well – praise indeed from him.

So what have I learned from this cancer journey of mine? I have learned that you forget about physical pain much more quickly than mental and emotional pain. I will never forget the mental anguish of seeing Jade escape from my arms and run towards a speeding van at age two (she stopped in time, thank God!). Nor will I forget the sadness and guilt of not getting to the nursing home in time on the day my father died. But I am already forgetting about the pain and discomfort of chemo and its side-effects – just like you forget the pain of childbirth. If, God forbid, I have to have chemo again in my life I will know exactly what to do and how to do it. I just hope that reading about my experiences and the advice I have been given will help cancer patients in the future; if that is the case, my job will be done.

I have learned to prioritise, to delegate and to say 'no'. Now I can justifiably be ruthless about dropping users and takers and avoiding negative people and situations!

I have learned that our children would rather have us alive and spending their inheritance than gone leaving them pots of money!

I have learned to be more patient, tolerant and grateful and I hope I have become a Better Person.

I have learned that all that requires deep breathing – inhale pure peach fresh air, exhale green bile. If that does not work, count to ten – slowly – then continue whatever you were doing that was annoying you.

And finally I have learned 'not to sweat the petty stuff and not to pet the sweaty stuff'!

I am so grateful to all the doctors, nurses, therapists, family and friends who between them have saved my life, 'My Left Boob' and my sanity. This is not the end; this is the afterwards. I am a Cancer Survivor and I am going to work hard to keep it that way.

Update, August 2013

In April 2013 Professor Smith tried Sally on Letrozole, supplemented by Calcichew.

In June Sally and Jade achieved their dream of swimming with the dolphins at Atlantis The Palm.

In July Sally was sadly diagnosed with secondary cancer. She is on oral chemo and once again fighting hard with her Marsden team, family, friends and the sterling Jade.

The sequel to this book will be published by Book Guild Publishing in 2014.

Alkalizing Foods

VEGETABLES

Alfalfa
Artichoke
Asparagus
Barley grass
Beets
Broccoli
Brussels sprouts
Cabbage
Carrot
Cauliflower
Celery
Chard
Chlorella
Collard greens
Corn, raw
Cucumber
Dandelion greens
Dulce
Edible flowers
Eggplant
Fermented veggies
Garlic
Kale
Kohlrabi
Lettuce
Mushrooms
Mustard greens
Nightshade veggies
Onions
Parsnips
Peas
Peppers
Pumpkin
Rutabaga
Sea veggies
Spinach
Spirulina
Squashes
String beans
Swiss chard
Watercress

Wheatgrass
Wild greens

RAW/COLD PRESSED OILS:

Almond, Avocado,
Coconut, Flaxseed,
Grapeseed, Hempseed,
MacNut, Olive

FRUITS

Apple
Apricot
Avocado
Banana
Berries
Cherries
Currants
Dates
Figs
Grapes
Grapefruit
Guava
Lemon
Lime
Mango
Melon
Nectarine
Orange
Peach
Pear
Persimmon
Pineapple
Plum
Pomegranate
Prunes
Raisins
Tangerine
Tomato

Tropical Fruits
Watermelon

PROTEIN

Almonds
Chestnuts
Millet
Seeds: Chia, Flax,
Pumpkin, Sunflower
Sprouted beans
Tempeh (fermented)
Tofu (fermented)

OTHER

Apple cider vinegar
Agar
Alkaline water
Banchi tea
Bee pollen
Dandelion tea
Fresh fruit juice
Ginseng tea
Green juices
Green tea
Herbal tea
Kombucha
Lecithin granules
Mineral water
Organic milk (raw/un-
pasteurised)
Probiotic cultures
Veggies juices
Young coconut water

SWEETENERS

Honey, raw and pure
Stevia

SPICES/
SEASONINGS

All herbs
Chilli pepper
Cinnamon
Curry powder
Ginger
Horseradish
Miso
Mustard

Sea Salt
Tamari and Coconut
aminos

ORIENTAL
VEGETABLES

Daikon
Dandelion root

Kelp
Kombu
Maitake
Nori
Reishi
Shitake
Umeboshi
Wakame

Acidifying Foods

NON-DAIRY FATS AND OILS (refined and processed)

Avocado oil
Canola oil
Corn oil
Hempseed oil
Lard
Olive oil
Safflower oil
Sesame oil
Sunflower oil

FRUITS

Cranberries

COOKED GRAINS

Amaranth
Barley
Buckwheat
Corn and products
Gluten
Hemp seed flour
Kamut
Oats (rolled)
Quinoa
Rice (all)
Rice cakes
Rye
Spelt
White flour
Whole wheat

DAIRY

Butter
Cheese, cow's milk
Cheese, goat's
Cheese, processed
Cheese, sheep's milk
Cottage cheese
Cream
Cream cheese
Ice cream
Margarine
Milk
Sour cream

SWEETENERS

Artificial sweeteners
Cane sugar
Corn syrup
Heated agave
Heated honey
Sorghum syrup

NUTS & BUTTERS

All roasted nuts
Brazil nuts
Cashews
Coconut, dried
Peanuts
Peanut butter
Pecans
Tahini
Walnuts

ANIMAL PROTEIN

All processed and
smoked meats
Beef
Carp
Clams
Egg yolks
Fish
Lamb
Lobster
Mussels
Oyster
Pork
Rabbit
Salmon
Scallops
Shrimp
Tuna
Turkey
Venison

PASTA (WHITE)

Macaroni
Noodles
Spaghetti

DRUGS & CHEMICALS

Chemicals
Drugs, medicinal
Herbicides
Pesticides
Tobacco

ALCOHOL

Beer
Spirits
Wine

BEANS & LEGUMES

Black beans
Green peas

Kidney beans
Lima beans
Pinto beans
Red beans
Soy beans
Soy – processed foods
White beans

OTHER

Braggs Liquid Aminos
Caffeine
Coffee
Distilled vinegar
Fried foods
Fruit juice, pasteurised
Potatoes

Processed/refined foods
Rice milk
Shortening
Soda
Soy milk
Table salt
Wheatgerm
Yeast and malt

NEUTRAL LEANING TO ALKALINE FOODS:

Adzuki beans
Almond milk
Amaranth
Black-eyed peas

Buckwheat
Chickpeas
Coconut
Cold-pressed safflower,
sesame, and sunflower
oil
Cottage cheese
Egg whites
Goat's milk cheese/
yogurt
Millet
Wild rice
Lentils
Macadamia nuts
Quinoa
Yogurt – unsweetened
Whey

Index